Current Topics in Neonatology Number 1

Current Topics in Neonatology Number 1

Edited by

Thomas N. Hansen
Chairman, Department of Pediatrics,
The Ohio State University,
Medical Director, Children's Hospital,
Columbus, Ohio, USA

and

Neil McIntosh
Department of Child Life and Health,
The University of Edinburgh,
Edinburgh,
Scotland, UK

W.B. SAUNDERS COMPANY LTD
London · Philadelphia · Toronto
Sydney · Tokyo

W.B. Saunders Company Ltd   24–28 Oval Road
London NW1 7DX, UK

The Curtis Center
Independence Square West
Philadelphia, PA 19106–3399, USA

Harcourt Brace & Company
55 Horner Avenue
Toronto, Ontario M8Z 4X6
Canada

Harcourt Brace & Company,
   Australia
30–52 Smidmore Street
Marrickville, NSW 2204, Australia

Harcourt Brace & Company, Japan
Ichibancho Central Building
22–1 Ichibancho
Chiyoda-ku, Tokyo 102, Japan

© 1996 W.B. Saunders Company Ltd

British Library Cataloguing in Publication Data is available

ISBN 0–7020–1980–1

This book is printed on acid-free paper

Typeset by Phoenix Photosetting, Chatham, Kent
Printed and bound in Great Britain by Biddles Ltd,
Guildford and King's Lynn

Contents

Contributors

Roberta A. Ballard Professor of Pediatrics, Obstetrics and Gynecology, University of Pennsylvania School of Medicine; Chief of Neonatology and Newborn Services, The Hospital of the University of Pennsylvania, The Children's Hospital of Philadelphia and 34th Street and Civic Centre Boulevard, Philadelphia, Pennsylvania 19104-4399, USA.

Hans-Ulrich Bucher Clinic for Neonatology, University Hospital, CH-8091 Zurich, Switzerland.

Annemarie Bucher-Schmid Clinic for Neonatology, University Hospital, CH-8091 Zurich, Switzerland.

Elizabeth A. Carse Consultant Neonatologist, Medical Co-ordinator, Growth and Development Clinic, Monash Medical Centre; Senior Lecturer, Department of Paediatrics, Monash University; Melbourne, Victoria, Australia.

Margaret P. Charlton Consultant Psychologist, Growth and Development Clinic, Monash Medical Centre, Melbourne, Victoria, Australia.

David A. Clark Professor of Pediatrics, Department of Pediatrics, LSU Medical School, 1542 Tulane Avenue, New Orleans, Louisiana 70112, USA.

Michael R. Gomez Neonatologist, Newborn Section of Pediatrics, Children's Clinic PA, Los Alamos Medical Center, Los Alamos, New Mexico, USA.

Anne Greenough Professor of Clinical Respiratory Physiology, Director of Neonatal and Paediatric Intensive Care Services, Department of Child Health, King's College Hospital, London SE5 9RS, UK.

Mark W. Kline   Associate Professor of Pediatrics, Sections of Allergy/Immunology and Infectious Diseases, Department of Pediatrics, Baylor College of Medicine and Texas Children's Hospital, Houston, Texas, USA.

Andrew J. Lyon   Consultant Neonatologist, Simpson Memorial Maternity Pavilion, Edinburgh EH3 9YW, UK.

Mark J.S. Miller   Research Professor in Pediatrics, Department of Pediatrics, LSU Medical School, 1542 Tulane Avenue, New Orleans, Louisiana 70112, USA.

Gunnar Sedin   Department of Paediatrics and Perinatal Research Laboratory, University Children's Hospital, S-751 85 Uppsala, Sweden.

John C. Sinclair   Departments of Pediatrics and of Clinical Epidemiology and Biostatistics, McMaster University Medical Centre, Department of Pediatrics, Room 4G4OC, 1200 Main Street West, Hamilton L8N 3ZS, Ontario, Canada.

Barbara Warner   Research Instructor of Pediatrics, University of Cincinnati College of Medicine, Division of Pulmonary Biology and Neonatology, Children's Hospital Medical Center, Cincinnati, Ohio, USA.

Jonathan Wispè   Associate Professor of Pediatrics, University of Cincinnati College of Medicine, Division of Pulmonary Biology and Neonatology, Children's Hospital Medical Center, Cincinnati, Ohio, USA.

John S. Wyatt   Reader in Neonatal Paediatrics, Department of Paediatrics, University College London Medical School, 5 University Street, London WC1E 6JJ, UK.

Victor Y.H. Yu   Director/Unit Head of Neonatal Intensive Care Unit and Growth and Development Clinic, Monash Medical Centre; Clinical Associate Professor, Department of Paediatrics, Monash University, Melbourne, Victoria, Australia.

Preface

Neonatal management in the areas of diagnosis and therapy continues to expand rapidly. Although the intricacies of special care are now well established, many elements of intensive care are questionable, or have become redundant as new techniques appear. Textbooks on neonatology are often largely out-of-date by the time they are published. *Current Topics in Neonatology* aims, on an annual basis, to provide up-to-date reviews of the rapidly changing areas of neonatology for clinicians working in this field. We hope to bring together expertise from both sides of the Atlantic, from the Antipodes and from elsewhere on the rapidly changing elements of care, so that busy practitioners may find useful state-of-the-art reviews, which can be used in conjunction with more formal neonatal volumes.

Thomas Hansen
Neil McIntosh

1

Genital Mycoplasmas and Infection in the Neonate

Andrew J. Lyon

INTRODUCTION

The organisms termed Mollicutes or Mycoplasmas were isolated over 50 years ago from the female lower genital tract[1,2] and subsequently from the human oropharynx[3]. Since then the number of species of Mycoplasmas and the range of diseases with which they have been associated has been ever increasing. *Mycoplasma hominis* and *Ureaplasma urealyticum* commonly inhabit the female urogenital tract and have been implicated in spontaneous abortion and premature onset of labour. These organisms have been isolated from several sites in the newborn preterm infant and have been associated with a range of diseases, including pneumonia, septicaemia, chronic lung disease, meningitis and hydrocephalus.

Most of the evidence linking the genital mycoplasmas to diseases of the newborn is from epidemiological studies, which, although suggesting an association, do not confirm cause and effect. Some of this work is convincing, however, and is supported by case reports showing a strong causal relationship between infection and disease. In particular there has been much interest in the possible role of *U. urealyticum* in the aetiology of chronic lung disease in the preterm infant. This review aims to summarize the evidence linking the genital mycoplasmas, and in particular *U. urealyticum*, with preterm delivery and disease in the newborn, to discuss possible mechanisms of action and to suggest guidelines for investigation and therapy.

THE MOLLICUTE FLORA OF HUMANS

More than 150 distinct species have been described within the class Mollicutes, including more than 92 *Mycoplasma* species found in humans, other animals and plants. These organisms are distinctive in lacking a cell wall. Ureaplasmas belong to this class and are distinguished from all other members of the order by the production of urease, giving them the ability to hydrolyse urea. The genus *Ureaplasma* contains a single species, *U. urealyticum*, with at least 14 different serotypes (or serovars).

M. *hominis* and *U. urealyticum* colonize the fetus in utero or at birth and are found in the oropharynx, lung and genital tract of newborns. The persistence of these two species declines after birth, but as many as 20% of prepubertal girls have the organisms in their lower genital tract. After puberty, genital colonization is related to sexual activity and reported rates vary from 40 to 80% of asymptomatic, sexually active women[4]. Isolation from other sites in the body, particularly the oropharynx, occurs rarely.

RELATIONSHIP TO PRETERM DELIVERY

Infection plays a major role in the aetiology of premature birth[5,6] and the frequent occurrence of the genital mycoplasmas in the female urogenital tract has raised interest in their possible role in preterm labour.

Colonization of the lower genital tract with *M. hominis* or *U. urealyticum* is more common in association with young maternal age, primigravidity, separated or single marital status, black race, low income, low educational status, high number of sexual partners, smoking, marijuana or cocaine use in pregnancy[7] and the presence of other genital organisms. These are all associated with an increased risk of preterm delivery and/or low birthweight and the importance of the mycoplasmas is difficult to unravel from these other related factors. A multicentre study involving 4934 women, evaluated for vaginal colonization with *U. urealyticum* at between 23 and 26 weeks gestation, failed to show any difference in pregnancy outcome between the colonized and non-colonized mothers when findings were adjusted for medical and sociodemographic factors[7]. Intervention studies aimed at eradicating the genital mycoplasmas from the lower genital tract have failed to prevent preterm labour or low birthweight[8], although erythromycin, the drug most commonly used in these studies, may be ineffective at the low pH in the vagina[4]. Overall there is little evidence that colonization of the vagina or cervix with these organisms is a cause of prematurity or low birthweight[9].

Invasion of the upper genital tract from ascending infection by a number of organisms, with the development of amnionitis and chorioamnionitis, has been clearly related to preterm delivery[10,11]. *U. urealyticum* has been isolated from amniotic fluid but, in contrast to other bacteria, this has not been significantly associated with prematurity[12]. This organism has been commonly isolated from the chorioamnion, being found in 38–66% of patients with histological chorioamnionitis compared with 13–17% of those without any microscopic changes[9], and could, therefore, be a possible cause of preterm labour. However, in all studies their presence has only been weakly associated with prematurity and this may be related to some other mechanism, such as a fetal or maternal immune response, or the action of other coexisting organisms. Further study on the relationship between these common organisms in the genital tract and prematurity is needed[9].

TRANSMISSION

Whether or not these organisms are responsible for the onset of preterm labour, there is no doubt that they are transmitted to the fetus and newborn baby. The vertical transmission rate for *U. urealyticum* ranges from nil to 55% among fullterm and from 29 to 55% in preterm infants born to infected mothers[13–15]. The organisms have been isolated from multiple sites but are most commonly found in the respiratory tract and vagina. Mode of delivery does not affect the colonization rate, but there is a significant increase in vertical transmission in the presence of chorioamnionitis or intra-amniotic infection[16]. Cassell et al reported that 14% of the *U. urealyticum* positive endotracheal aspirates collected within 24 hours of birth, in infants of birthweight <2500 g, were from those delivered by caesarean section with intact membranes[17], suggesting that the organism is capable of crossing the placenta or the membranes are not a barrier. The infant colonization rate within a given population will depend on the prevalence of maternal carriage but, in all, it appears to be higher in the very low birthweight infants. In one study the vertical transmission rate was 89% in infants below 1000 g compared with 54% in those above this birthweight[14]. This correlates with the increased isolation of *U. urealyticum* from the chorioamnion in very low birthweight infants, the rate being almost three times higher than in those born with a birthweight >1500 g[5].

The infant can, therefore, acquire these organisms either in utero, after haematogenous spread or inhalation of infected amniotic fluid, or during delivery through an infected birth canal with colonization of skin, mucosa and respiratory tract. Whether nosocomial transmission can occur after birth is uncertain. In the neonatal period, Sanchez and Regan reported that in those babies found to have *U. urealyticum* 89% were positive by the end of the first week of life, 8% by the second and 3% in the fourth week[14], results similar to those in a study by Lyon et al[18]. A possible explanation for these findings is that the infants were infected after birth following nosocomial transmission. There is, however, no further evidence that these organisms are capable of infecting infants after birth[19], but that colonization or infection appears only later in association with sexual activity. Some babies may appear to become positive at some time after birth because of the difficulties in culturing these organisms, which may only appear in large numbers once the microflora of the infant has been altered by the broad spectrum antibiotics commonly used in neonatal units. More work with sensitive methods of detection, such as the polymerase chain reaction, and specific serotyping of isolates is needed to confirm whether nosocomial transmission in the neonate is of importance.

Colonization of the newborn with *U. urealyticum* is usually transient, with isolation rates decreasing after 3 months of age, although preterm infants can carry the organism in their respiratory tract for several months[17].

INFECTION IN THE NEONATE

The finding of the genital mycoplasmas in every organ system, including the bloodstream, of the fetus and neonate has generated much interest in their potential as pathogens capable of causing disseminated infection[20].

Bloodstream Infections

U. urealyticum has been found in blood cultures from infants in whom the organism has been isolated from endotracheal secretions[17] and in those with definite pneumonia[21,22]. It is not known how often *U. urealyticum* in the bloodstream of neonates causes significant illness, although it should be considered as a possible pathogen, particularly in the preterm infant.

Central Nervous System Infections

The finding of the genital mycoplasmas in the bloodstream has raised the possibility that they may be implicated in central nervous system (CNS) infections. In two studies in different hospitals, Waites et al reported positive cerebrospinal fluid (CSF) cultures for *U. urealyticum* or *M. hominis* in 13/100[23] and 14/318[24] preterm infants.

Particular care was taken to avoid contamination from the skin, although the possibility that some positive cultures could have been due to blood from a traumatic tap cannot be excluded. However, there were several isolates from CSF that contained no red cells. Shaw et al dispute the importance of *U. urealyticum* as a significant cause of meningitis, finding only one positive CSF culture in a prospective study of 135 preterm infants, although the indication for lumbar puncture was not stated[25]. Others have also failed to isolate mycoplasmas from CSF but many of these studies included mainly older infants in whom infection with these organisms is less likely[26].

U. urealyticum has been isolated from CSF in infants with intraventricular haemorrhage and from those with hydrocephalus. In at least half the reported cases the organism was also isolated from the lower respiratory tract, raising the possibility that this was the source of the CNS infection. Possible sequestration in large intraventricular clots with persistence of the organism over several weeks has been reported[27]. A convincing piece of evidence that these organisms have the potential to cause serious CNS disease is the production of meningitis and hydrocephalus in newborn mice and beagles using pure cultures of *U. urealyticum* isolated from the CSF of human infants[4].

Little is known about the natural history, epidemiology and prognosis of systemic mycoplasma diseases and their importance in CNS infection, with information limited to individual reports. Infants have been described with either a subclinical illness or a complete recovery following mild disease. Reduction in hydrocephalus after treatment has been documented and in one study 50% of the ureaplasma infected infants died soon after identification of the CSF infection[27]. More prospective studies are needed to define the place of these organisms in systemic and CNS infections in the newborn.

Waites et al[27] suggest that a mycoplasma aetiology be considered in any infant with CSF pleocytosis who has negative Gram stains and/or bacterial cultures, as well as those with progressive hydrocephalus, although Shaw et al[25] would argue against the need for such routine investigation. The incidence of meningitis is greater in the neonatal period than during any other period of life. Many lumbar punctures are done but positive bacterial cultures in CSF are rare. The prevalence of mycoplasmas in the preterm population is high enough to make it advisable to consider them in the sick infant with suspected CNS infection, particularly in the presence of a white cell response in the CSF and negative bacterial cultures.

Respiratory Infections

Respiratory disease is the most common cause of perinatal mortality and morbidity. It is the possible role of the genital mycoplasmas in the aetiology of the lung problems of the preterm baby that has generated most interest in recent years.

Neonatal pneumonia

U. urealyticum has been shown to cause pneumonia[28] and has been associated with persistent pulmonary hypertension in the newborn[21]. The organism has been isolated from the lungs of newborns with pneumonia and these isolates produce pneumonic changes when inoculated into newborn animals[29,30].

Ollikainen et al studied the early respiratory problems in infants <34 weeks gestation who were colonized with U. urealyticum and compared them with those not infected[31]. Respiratory distress syndrome, the need for assisted ventilation, severe respiratory insufficiency and death were significantly more common among infected infants. They concluded that U. urealyticum infection was associated with an unfavourable short term outcome in preterm infants, although the exact mechanism for this was not known. This study included infants up to 33 weeks gestation and many would be expected to have only minimal lung problems – only 35 of the 98 studied were given surfactant. The infected group had a lower gestation and a greater male preponderance than the non-infected, both factors which would be expected to produce a poorer outcome. No information was given about the use of antenatal steroids in the mothers. Crouse et al[32] showed that in infants of birthweight ≤1250 g, those infected with *U. urealyticum* had radiographic evidence of more severe pulmonary disease, with evidence of pneumonia and early changes of bronchopulmonary dysplasia, compared with similar non-infected babies. These differences were independent of prematurity, race and sex.

Despite many criticisms of these studies, there is now a body of evidence that points to *U. urealyticum*, and possibly also *M. hominis*, being a significant pathogen in the respiratory tract of some preterm infants, particularly those with a birthweight below 1250 g. However, their overall importance in the aetiology of early lung disease and the role of specific antibiotic treatment needs further study.

Chronic lung disease

Chronic lung disease (CLD) is a persisting problem among preterm survivors and its incidence has not declined despite improvements in neonatal care[33]. The aetiology of CLD is multifactorial, with gestation and positive pressure ventilation being the most important factors. The literature on the association between infection of the lower respiratory tract with *U. urealyticum* and CLD is extensive, although a definite cause and effect relationship has never been proven. Interpretation of a whole host of studies is complicated by differences in design, definitions of CLD, patient populations, methods of specimen collection and neonatal management.

Sanchez and Regan[34] report a 30% incidence of bronchopulmonary dysplasia among infants weighing <2000 g colonized with *U. urealyticum*, compared with 8% in those not colonized. This study used pharyngeal cultures and the results are difficult to interpret as there is a poor correlation between these isolates and those obtained from endotracheal aspiration[17].

Wang et al[35] found CLD in 51% of infants weighing <1250 g who were colonized with *U. urealyticum* in gastric, nasopharyngeal or tracheal aspirates, compared with 16% in those without the organism. They did not rule out other concomitant bacterial infections that may have contributed to lung disease.

Cassell et al[17] isolated *U. urealyticum* from 17% of endotracheal aspirates obtained within the first day of life from 200 infants with respiratory distress and who weighed <2500 g. Another 10% were positive for *M. hominis* and these two organisms were the most commonly isolated. CLD occurred in 82% of infants weighing ≤1000 g who were positive for *U. urealyticum*, compared with 41% of those with negative cultures ($P < 0.02$), and in this weight group death was twice as likely if the baby was infected. There was no association between infection and CLD or death in infants with birthweight >1000 g.

There has been a critical review of four recent independent studies linking *U. urealyticum* and CLD[36], including the three mentioned above[17,34,35,37]. All showed a significant association between ureaplasma colonization of the respiratory tract in the first 3 days of life and the development of CLD in very low birthweight infants. Despite differences in study design the relative risks of developing CLD in colonized infants were very similar, and those infected did not differ from the non-infected in respect of other aetiological factors for CLD. A closer look at birthweight groups showed a significantly increased risk of CLD in infected infants with a birthweight <1250 g, which was not seen in those above this weight. In only one of the studies were the infants treated with surfactant[37] but this did not appear to have any impact on the incidence of CLD or on the differences between infected and non-infected infants. Surfactant has been shown to have an effect on multiplication of the group B streptococcus in the airways[38] and a recent report found that Survanta, derived from cow lungs, but not Exosurf, a synthetic surfactant, inhibited the growth of *U. urealyticum*[39]. This possible inhibitory effect will need to be considered in any future work into the place of these organisms in the aetiology of lung disease in preterm infants.

It appears that only the very low birthweight infants are susceptible to disease with the genital mycoplasmas. This may account for some of the disparities among earlier studies on the role of *U. urealyticum* in neonatal lung disease, which failed to distinguish this high risk population.

Not all workers have found an association between the genital mycoplasmas and CLD. Saxen et al[40] studied ventilated babies <30 weeks gestation in Finland and reported a 31% infection rate for *U. urealyticum* or *M. hominis*. Forty-three per cent of the infected babies developed CLD, compared with 29% of the non-infected, a difference which was not significant. Smyth et al[41], reporting on ventilated infants with a birthweight <1500 g, found only 13% to be culture positive for *U. urealyticum*. Of the infected babies, 78% developed CLD, compared with 54% of the non-infected, and logistic regression analysis revealed early gestation, but not mycoplasma colonization, to be independently associated with CLD. The infection rate was lower than in many other studies and as a result the numbers in the infected group were small.

CLD is most commonly defined as continuing oxygen dependence at 28 days in a baby who has been ventilated and who has abnormal chest radiograph changes, but this correlates poorly with long term outcome. Many extremely low birthweight infants will still be in oxygen at 28 days and may have persistent radiographic changes, yet do not go on to develop classical CLD. Better correlation with long term outcome is obtained if CLD is defined as oxygen dependence at 36 weeks equivalent gestation[42]. Lyon et al[18] reported positive cultures of *U. urealyticum* or *M. hominis* in 30% of tracheal aspirates in ventilated babies ≤30 weeks gestation, and CLD, defined as oxygen dependence at 36 weeks gestation, was found in 90% of the infected and 50% of the non-infected babies ($P<0.01$). It would be interesting to know if, in the negative studies by Saxen et al[40] and Smyth et al[41], there was still no difference in incidence of CLD between the infected and non-infected groups at 36 weeks.

The evidence for the association between these organisms and CLD in the preterm infant is compelling, particularly from the careful studies by Cassell et al, but we still lack any definite proof of a cause and effect relationship.

MECHANISMS OF ACTION

If these organisms are capable of causing lung disease in preterm infants, are there any clues to the mechanism of their action?

Cassell et al[17] speculated that damage was due to a chronic subclinical pulmonary infection, resulting in prolonged respiratory support and resultant lung injury. *U. urealyticum* has been shown to cause pneumonia, and in cell culture can induce both cellular necrosis and ciliary injury in human fetal tracheal cultures by the production of ammonium ions[43].

The 140 day gestation baboon is an established model for prematurity[44], developing the same physiological and pathological characteristics as human neonates of 30–32 weeks gestation. Walsh et al[30] introduced *U. urealyticum* into the trachea of three of these animals, all of which had respiratory distress syndrome similar to that of the human. After 6 days of ventilation all three grew *U. urealyticum* from lung tissue and all had epithelial ulceration of the airways with marked neutrophil infiltration. This acute inflammatory response was not seen in four uninfected control animals.

The ability of *U. urealyticum* to cause pneumonia in humans and the findings in cell culture and animal models suggest that stimulation of the inflammatory response may be important in the patho-genesis of any long term damage these organisms may cause. High white cell counts have been found in preterm infants colonized with *U. urealyticum* in whom no other organisms were cultured, suggesting that the mycoplasma is capable of eliciting an inflammatory reaction and may be a true pathogen in the neonate[45]. *U. urealyticum* is capable of inducing an immunological response, which suggests it is more than just a benign colonizing organism. IgA reactive to *U. urealyticum* has been detected in cord blood and has been more commonly found in infants <30 weeks gestation compared with those more mature[46]. Quinn et al[47] have shown the production of serovar specific IgG and IgM to *U. urealyticum* and elevated levels of these antibodies were associated with a higher mortality among neonates with respiratory disease. Patients with hypogammaglobulinaemia have been found to be at risk of invasive disease from these organisms[48]. This suggests that antibody is important for protection and may in part explain the apparent increased susceptibility of the more immature babies below 30 weeks gestation[17,49].

The role of inflammatory mediators in the pathogenesis of lung damage is of current interest. The alveolar macrophage appears to be the key cell both in the normal defence of the lung and in damaging processes[50]. The α-chemokine interleukin 8 (IL-8) is produced by this cell, and by lung fibroblasts, in response to a number of insults, including bacterial products and hyperoxia. IL-8 attracts and acti-vates polymorphs as well as stimulating the alveolar macrophage to produce other cytokines, in particular tumour necrosis factor α (TNF-α) which appears to be of prime importance in pulmonary pathophysiology. The overall picture is complex, with no study yet able to elucidate the exact way in which the inflammatory mediators interact in the lung of the preterm infant or how the processes develop with time. All studies measure the cytokines in fluid obtained by bronchoalveolar lavage and relate the responses in the first few days of life to a chronic lung condition that develops over several weeks. Trying to follow the inflammatory changes over long periods of time is difficult because the control group, who do not develop CLD, tend to be extubated after only a few days, making further bronchoalveolar lavage impossible. However, in the first days of life neonates at risk for the development of CLD show an enhanced inflammatory reaction in the lungs, with an increased production of a number of mediators, and an associated increase in pulmonary microvascular permeability[51]. High levels of IL-8 have been found in the early stages of respiratory distress syndrome and may be of prognostic significance for the development of CLD[52]. TNF-α is important in the normal defences of the body, but excess production, which may be harmful, has been documented in both adult and neonatal respiratory distress syndrome[53]. Persistence of these and other mediators may be due to the preterm infant's inability to downregulate the normal inflammatory response, which then, instead of protecting, damages the lung[54]. If this hypothesis is confirmed in further work, it will make therapeutic sense to attempt to block the inflammatory process as far 'upstream' as possible and target the production of the early mediators such as IL-8 and TNF-α[53].

If the inflammatory mediators are responsible for chronic lung damage, is there any evidence that the genital mycoplasmas could be responsible for triggering this response? Stancombe et al[55] have shown that human neonatal fibroblasts release significant amounts of IL-6 and IL-8 in direct response to infection with *U. urealyticum*, the levels of these cytokines being higher than from cells exposed to oxygen alone or to lipopolysaccharide. Groneck et al[56] found significantly higher levels of a number of inflammatory mediators, including IL-8, in the trachea of infants of birthweight <1200 g colonized with *U. urealyticum* compared with those not colonized. The inflammation was not found beyond day 10 of life and they postulated that this was related to clearance of the organism from the airways, although this was not confirmed by culture data. This study concluded that *U. urealyticum* was not a causative agent for CLD in general, although persistent infection in some babies may be an aetiological factor.

The finding of high levels, in vitro and in vivo, of the early mediators of the inflammatory response in the presence of *U. urealyticum*, along with the histological lesions found in the baboon, suggests that this organism is capable of acute inflammatory damage to the airways. The question is whether this early response is of any real significance and can go on to cause chronic lung damage. Groneck et al[56] demonstrated a fall in IL-8 and TNF-α over the first week of life and this appears to be the general pattern for these early mediators[52]. However, it is possible that other markers further down the inflammatory cascade may be present in high levels and contribute to ongoing damage, although no one as yet has been able to quantify these as a cause of lung pathology.

A variability in the immune response, combined with differences in serovar pathogenicity and genetic predisposition of the infant, may explain why not all infants colonized with the genital mycoplasmas develop chronic lung disease[28,57]. Another explanation for the variation in response to these organisms may be that a cofactor is needed before significant pulmonary damage occurs. The aetiology of CLD is multifactorial and in any individual baby many factors will be present at any one time. Oxygen is of particular importance, and newborn mice infected with *U. urealyticum* have longer periods of infectivity and a higher mortality in the presence of hyperoxia, when compared with those exposed to either oxygen or infection alone[58]. It is possible that subclinical pulmonary inflammation due to mycoplasma infection results in the need for prolonged respiratory support, leading to oxygen-induced lung injury. This condition may interfere with the pulmonary defence mechanisms, promoting further injury by other pathogenic organisms. This theory is supported by the observation that oxidants can enhance susceptibility to infectious lung diseases, and in particular to other respiratory disease due to mycoplasmas[59]. In rabbits, however, although hyperoxia caused a significant inflammatory response, this was not exacerbated by infection with *U. urealyticum*[60], but in this study the animals were only exposed to oxygen for 24 hours.

DETECTION

The genital mycoplasmas can be cultured in liquid specimens, including blood, amniotic fluid, CSF, urine, pleural fluid and tracheobronchial secretions. They are susceptible to fluctuations in environmental conditions, particularly drying and osmotic changes. Specimens should not be allowed to sit at room temperature but be either stored at 4°C in a sealed container or inoculated into a specific transport medium. The organisms are stable for long periods when frozen at −70°C in a protein-containing support medium. Ureaplasmas are unique in producing a urease that splits urea and causes a pH shift in the culture broth, a reaction that can be detected as a colour change and used as an indicator of growth. Broth cultures showing such a change can then be subcultured on agar under 5% CO_2[4].

Successful culture of these organisms requires special expertise and is costly, taking at least 3–5 days to get a result. The polymerase chain reaction has been used to detect both *U. urealyticum* and *M. hominis* and may be a more sensitive, as well as a faster, technique than bacterial culture[61,62]. There have been problems with inhibitors, probably polypeptides, to the DNA amplification in the endotracheal aspirates from preterm infants but these can be overcome by altering the dilution of the specimen and by addition of increasing amounts of a proteinase to the solution[61].

The production of IgA and serovar specific IgM and IgG are indicative of infection with these organisms and are important in protection. Apart from the finding by Quinn et al[47], that mortality was higher among neonates with elevated antibodies and respiratory disease, the relationship between the immune response and disease has not been clarified.

TREATMENT

The genital mycoplasmas, and in particular *U. urealyticum*, can cause invasive disease in some preterm infants, although it is by no means clear which are at most risk. Their place in the aetiology of CLD is still controversial. They are also commonly found in many healthy individuals, and it is difficult to establish guidelines for recognition and management of clinically significant conditions due to these organisms. Screening of all neonates for *U. urealyticum* and *M. hominis* is not justified but should be considered in those with clinical evidence of infection, particularly when no other organism has been identified or if there is a failure to respond to broad spectrum antibiotics. They are among the most common organisms isolated from the CSF and must be considered in neonates with unexplained CSF pleocytosis. It is important when considering the possibility of respiratory disease that endotracheal secretions are cultured because nasopharyngeal aspirates or gastric washings do not reflect the status of the lung itself[17].

As these organisms lack a cell wall they are not affected by β-lactam antibiotics and their failure to synthesize folic acid makes them resistant to sulphonamides or trimethoprim. They are generally susceptible to drugs that interfere with protein synthesis, such as tetracycline and macrolides. Most other antibiotics used routinely in neonatal intensive care have little effect, except possibly gentamicin, which may have some activity against these organisms. The therapeutic options are well reviewed by Waites et al[63]. Resistance to both tetracycline[64] and erythromycin[65] has been reported for *U. urealyticum*. Despite this, for over 90% of the strains, erythromycin is the most promising currently available antimicrobial agent and has been shown to eradicate the organism from the lower respiratory tract of the preterm newborn[66]. Penetration of erythromycin into the CSF is poor and, in infants deteriorating with evidence of meningitis, tetracycline is probably more effective. *M. hominis* has a high incidence of resistance to erythromycin[67]. The place of this organism in acute disease of the neonate is less well studied and recommendations about the need for treatment and which antibiotic to use cannot be made on current knowledge.

As well as its antibacterial activity, erythromycin has been found to have anti-inflammatory properties. In adults with respiratory disease this drug reduced the neutrophil count and activity[68] as well as the production of IL-8[69] in bronchoalveolar secretions. The relative importance of this anti-inflammatory action has not been elucidated.

The optimum treatment schedule for *U. urealyticum* with erythromycin is not known. Eradication in the lower respiratory tract has been demonstrated with treatment for at least 7 days[66] but whether this is permanent or whether the organisms can reappear after therapy stops is not certain. Limited clinical experience and pharmacokinetic data suggest a 10–14 day course for infants without CSF involvement, using 25–40 mg kg^{-1} day^{-1} of erythromycin lactobionate in three or four divided doses. This schedule achieves drug levels that exceed the minimum inhibitory concentration for *U. urealyticum*[66]. Even the organisms that show some resistance to erythromycin can be eradicated with this treatment, possibly because the concentration of the drug in pulmonary secretions may exceed that in serum[70]. In CNS infections it would seem reasonable to start with erythromycin and monitor both clinical progress and whether the organism is eradicated from the CSF. There are no guidelines as to length of treatment but failure to respond or a deteriorating condition should prompt a change to a tetracycline. Shaw et al[25] described an infant from whom *U. urealyticum* was persistently isolated from CSF over 16 weeks despite a protracted course of erythromycin. Eradication was finally achieved with doxycycline.

There are no data on the relative efficacy of the intravenous versus the oral route for erythromycin in the preterm infant. In term infants the serum levels of the drug after intravenous infusion have not been found to be significantly different from those achieved by the oral route[71]. The problem is whether these data can be extrapolated to the preterm infant with its differences in body composition, drug distribution, protein binding and hepatic and renal excretion. At present, in significant infections in the preterm infant, the intravenous route is recommended, although erythromycin has to be given by infusion over 30–60 minutes and can be irritant to the veins. There is nothing so far to suggest that intravenous erythromycin is unsafe in the preterm newborn, and, in particular, there is no evidence of ototoxicity[70,72], a problem reported in adults with impaired renal and/or hepatic function[73]. In older children the concurrent administration of theophylline or caffeine with erythromycin may be associated with an increase in serum theophylline levels and possible toxicity. The magnitude of this problem in the neonate has not been evaluated but in this situation it would be prudent to monitor theophylline levels closely.

CONCLUSIONS

The genital mycoplasmas are common organisms in the female lower genital tract and ascending infection may be implicated in the aetiology of preterm labour. They are found in many sites in the newborn infant and vertical transmission from infected mothers is common. *U. urealyticum* has been the most widely studied and is capable of causing inflammation in the very low birthweight infant. Failure of the preterm newborn to control and downregulate the inflammatory response may result in a process, which, although initially protective, with persistence becomes increasingly damaging. Erythromycin can eradicate *U. urealyticum* at least transiently from the respiratory tract but further studies are needed to determine not only if this is permanent but also whether there is any real clinical benefit to routine treatment for these common organisms. *U. urealyticum* is capable of invasive disease and, with the present state of our knowledge, it makes sense to consider it in preterm infants with evidence of infection where bacterial cultures are consistently negative.

CLD remains a challenge because of its continued prevalence in the preterm survivor despite advances in neonatal care. Investigation into the contribution of multiple factors, such as infection with *U. urealyticum* or other organisms, to CLD is needed, and a placebo controlled trial of erythromycin treatment of colonized neonates may help assess causality. Such a study may not fully explain the relationship between ureaplasma infection and CLD if there are other organisms that are inhibited by erythromycin, or if treatment fails to eradicate *U. urealyticum*. The apparent anti-inflammatory properties of the drug itself may also have a direct effect and prove to be of importance. It may be that, even if infection is a factor in the aetiology of CLD, it will be more effective to modulate the immune response, at an early stage, with steroids or other anti-inflammatory drugs, rather than treat with antibiotics.

REFERENCES

1. Dienes L and Edsall G. Observations on the L-organism of Klieneberger. *Proc Soc Exp Biol Med* 1937;**36:**740–744.
2. Dienes L. Cultivation of pleuropneumonia-like organisms from female genital organs. *Proc Soc Exp Biol Med* 1940;**44:**468–469.
3. Smith PF and Morton HE. Isolation of pleuropneumonia-like organisms from the throats of humans. *Science* 1951;**113:**623–624.
4. Cassell GH, Waites KB, Watson H-L, Crouse DT and Harasawa R. *Ureaplasma urealyticum* intrauterine infections: role in prematurity and disease in newborns. *Clin Microbiol Rev* 1993;**6:**69–87.
5. Hillier SL, Martius M, Krohn M, Kiviat N, Holmes KK and Eschenbach DA. A case–control study of chorioamniotic infection and histologic chorioamnionitis in prematurity. *N Engl J Med* 1988;**319:**972–978.
6. Hay PE, Lamont RF, Taylor-Robinson D, Morgan DJ, Ison C and Pearson J. Abnormal bacterial colonisation of the genital tract and subsequent preterm delivery and late miscarriage. *BMJ* 1984;**308:**295–298.
7. Carey JC, Blackwelder WC, Nugent RP et al. Antepartum cultures for *Ureaplasma urealyticum* are not useful in predicting pregnancy outcome. *Am J Obstet Gynecol* 1991;**164:**728–733.
8. Eschenbach DA, Nugent RP, Rao AV et al. A randomized placebo-controlled trial of erythromycin for the treatment of *Ureaplasma urealyticum* to prevent premature labour. *Am J Obstet Gynecol* 1991;**164:**734–742.
9. Eschenbach DA. *Ureaplasma urealyticum* and premature birth. *Clin Infect Dis* 1993;**17(suppl. 1):**S100–106.
10. Gibbs RS, Romero R, Hillier SL, Eschenbach DA and Sweet RL. A review of premature birth and subclinical infection. *Am J Obstet Gynecol* 1992;**166:**1515–1528.
11. Watts DH, Krohn MA, Hillier SL and Eschenbach DA. The association of occult amniotic fluid infection with gestational age and neonatal outcome among women in preterm labour. *Obstet Gynecol* 1992;**79:**351–357.
12. Zlatnik FJ, Gellhaus TM, Benda JA, Koontz FP and Burmeister LF. Histologic chorioamnionitis, microbial infection and prematurity. *Obstet Gynecol* 1990;**76:**355–359.
13. Sanchez PJ and Regan JA. Vertical transmission of *Ureaplasma urealyticum* in full term infants. *Pediatr Infect Dis J* 1987;**6:**825–828.
14. Sanchez PJ and Regan JA. Vertical transmission of *Ureaplasma urealyticum* from mothers to preterm infants. *Pediatr Infect Dis J* 1990;**9:**398–401.
15. Horowitz S, Landau D, Shinwell ES, Zmora E and Dagan R. Respiratory tract colonization with *Ureaplasma urealyticum* and bronchopulmonary dysplasia in neonates in southern Israel. *Pediatr Infect Dis J* 1992;**11:**847–851.
16. Dinsmoor MJ, Ramamurthy RS and Gibbs RS. Transmission of genital mycoplasmas from mother to neonate in women with prolonged membrane rupture. *Pediatr Infect Dis J* 1989;**8:**483–487.
17. Cassell GH, Waites KB, Crouse DT et al. Association of *Ureaplasma urea-*

lyticum infection of the lower respiratory tract with chronic lung disease and death in very-low-birth-weight infants. *Lancet* 1988;**ii:**240–245.

18. Lyon AJ, Iles R, Ross P and McIntosh N. Urogenital mycoplasmas in neonatal endotracheal secretions and the development of chronic lung disease (CLD). *Pediatr Res* 1994;**36(part 2):**19 (abstract).

19. Litiknukal S, Kusmiesz H, Nelson JD and McCracken GH Jr. Role of genital mycoplasmas in young infants with suspected sepsis. *J Pediatr* 1986;**109:**971–974.

20. Cassell GH, Waites KB, Gibbs RS and Davis JK. Role of *Ureaplasma urealyticum* in amnionitis. *Pediatr Infect Dis J* 1986;**5(suppl.):**S247–252.

21. Waites KB, Crouse DT, Philips JB III, Canupp KC and Cassell GH. Ureaplasmal pneumonia and sepsis associated with persistent pulmonary hypertension of the newborn. *Pediatrics* 1989;**83:**79–85.

22. Brus F, van Waarde WM, Schoots C and Oetomo SB. Fatal ureaplasma pneumonia and sepsis in a newborn infant. *Eur J Pediatr* 1991; **150:**782–783.

23. Waites KB, Rudd PT, Crouse DT et al. Chronic *Ureaplasma urealyticum* and *Mycoplasma hominis* infections of central nervous system in preterm infants. *Lancet* 1988;**i:**17–21.

24. Waites KB, Duffy LB, Crouse DT et al. Mycoplasmal infections of cerebrospinal fluid in newborn infants from a community hospital population. *Pediatr Infect Dis J* 1990;**9:**241–245.

25. Shaw NJ, Pratt BC and Weindling AM. Ureaplasma and mycoplasma infections of the central nervous system in preterm infants. *Lancet* 1989;**ii:**1530–1531.

26. Likitnukul S, Nelson JD, McCracken GH and Kusmiesz H. Rarity of genital mycoplasmas in young infants with aseptic meningitis. *J Pediatr* 1987;**110:**998.

27. Waites KB, Crouse DT and Cassell GH. Systemic neonatal infection due to *Ureaplasma urealyticum*. *Clin Infect Dis* 1993;**17(suppl. 1):**S131–135.

28. Cassell GH, Waites KB and Crouse DT. Perinatal mycoplasmal infections. *Clin Perinatol* 1991;**18:**241–262.

29. Rudd PT, Cassell GH, Waites KB, Davis JK and Duffy LB. Experimental production of *Ureaplasma urealyticum* pneumonia and demonstration of age-related susceptibility. *Infect Immun* 1989;**57:**818–825.

30. Walsh WF, Butler J, Coalson J, Hensley D, Cassell GH and deLemos RA. A primate model of *Ureaplasma urealyticum* in the premature infant with hyaline membrane disease. *Clin Infect Dis* 1993;**17(suppl.):**S158–162.

31. Ollikainen J, Hiekkaniemi H, Korppi M, Sarkkinen H and Heinonen K. *Ureaplasma urealyticum* infection associated with acute respiratory insufficiency and death in premature infants. *J Pediatr* 1993;**122:**756–760.

32. Crouse DT, Odrezin GT, Cutter GR et al. Radiographic changes associated with tracheal isolation of *Ureaplasma urealyticum* from neonates. *Clin Infect Dis* 1993;**17(suppl.):**S122–130.

33. Northway WH. Bronchopulmonary dysplasia: then and now. *Arch Dis Child* 1990;**65:**1076–1081.

34. Sanchez PJ and Regan JA. *Ureaplasma urealyticum* colonization and chronic lung disease in very low birth weight infants. *Pediatr Infect Dis J* 1988;7:542–546.

35. Wang EE, Frayha H, Watts J et al. The role of *Ureaplasma urealyticum* and other pathogens in the development of chronic lung disease of prematurity. *Pediatr Infect Dis J* 1988;7:547–551.

36. Wang EEL, Cassell GH, Sanchez PJ, Regan JA, Payne NR and Liu PP. *Ureaplasma urealyticum* and chronic lung disease of prematurity: critical appraisal of the literature on causation. *Clin Infect Dis* 1993; 17(suppl.):S112–116.

37. Payne NR, Steinberg S, Ackerman P, Chrenka BA, Sane S and Anderson KT. New prospective studies of association of *Ureaplasma urealyticum* colonization and chronic lung disease. *Clin Infect Dis* 1993; 17(suppl.):S117–121.

38. Sherman MP, Campbell LA, Merritt TA et al. Effect of different surfactants on pulmonary group B streptococcal infection in premature rabbits. *J Pediatr* 1994;125:939–947.

39. Walsh WF, Hensley D and Greenberg D. Effect of surfactant on *Ureaplasma urealyticum* growth. *Pediatr Res* 1994;35(part 2):305 (abstract).

40. Saxen H, Hakkarainen K, Pohjavuori M and Miettinen A. Chronic lung disease of preterm infants in Finland is not associated with *Ureaplasma urealyticum* colonization. *Acta Paediatr* 1993;82:198–201.

41. Smyth AR, Shaw NJ, Pratt BC and Weindling AM. Ureaplasma urealyticum and chronic lung disease. *Eur J Pediatr* 1993;152:931–932.

42. Shennan AT, Dunn MS, Ohlsson A, Lennox K and Hoskins EM. Abnormal pulmonary outcomes in premature infants: prediction from oxygen requirements in the neonatal period. *Pediatrics* 1988;82:527–532.

43. Quinn PA, Gilan JE, Markstad D et al. Intrauterine infection with *Ureaplasma urealyticum* as a cause of fatal neonatal pneumonia. *Pediatr Infect Dis J* 1985;4:538–543.

44. Escobedo MB, Hilliard JL, Smith F et al. A baboon model of bronchopulmonary dysplasia. 1. Clinical features. *Exp Mol Pathol* 1982;37:323–324.

45. Ohlsson A, Wang E and Vearncombe M. Leukocyte counts and colonization with *Ureaplasma urealyticum* in preterm neonates. *Clin Infect Dis* 1993;17(suppl.):S144–147.

46. Cunningham C, Bonville C, Belkowitz J and Weiner L. IgA reactivity to *Ureaplasma urealyticum*: immunoblot analysis of cord blood samples. *Pediatr Res* 1994;35(part 2):296 (abstract).

47. Quinn PA, Li HCS, Th'ng C, Dunn M and Butnay J. Serological response to *Ureaplasma urealyticum* in the neonate. *Clin Infect Dis* 1993; 17(suppl.):S136–143.

48. Taylor-Robinson D, Furr PM and Webster ADB. *Ureaplasma urealyticum* in the immunocompromised host. *Pediatr Infect Dis J* 1986;5:S236–238.

49. Cassell GH, Crouse DT, Waites KB, Rudd PT and Davis JK. Does *Ureaplasma urealyticum* cause respiratory disease in the newborn? *Pediatr Infect Dis J* 1988;7:535–541.

50. Murch SH. Cellular mediators of lung damage. *Br J Intensive Care* 1995;**5**:27–32.

51. Groneck P, Götze-Speer B, Oppermann M, Eiffert H and Speer CP. Association of pulmonary inflammation and increased microvascular permeability during the development of bronchopulmonary dysplasia: a sequential analysis of inflammatory mediators in respiratory fluids of high-risk preterm neonates. *Pediatrics* 1994;**93**:712–718.

52. McColm J and McIntosh N. Interleukin-8 in bronchoalveolar secretions as predictor of chronic lung disease in premature infants. *Lancet* 1994;**343**:729.

53. Murch SH, MacDonald IT, Wood CBS and Costeloe KL. Tumour necrosis factor in bronchoalveolar secretions of infants with the respiratory distress syndrome and the effect of dexamethasone treatment. *Thorax* 1992;**47**:44–47.

54. Bagchi A, Viscardi RM, Taciak V, Ensor JE, McCrea KA and Hasday JD. Increased activity of interleukin-6 but not tumour necrosis factor-α in lung lavage of premature infants is associated with the development of bronchopulmonary dysplasia. *Pediatr Res* 1994;**36**:244–252.

55. Stancombe BB, Walsh WF, Derdak S, Dixon P and Hensley D. Induction of human pulmonary fibroblast cytokines by hyperoxia and *Ureaplasma urealyticum*. *Clin Infect Dis* 1993;**17(suppl.)**:S154–157.

56. Groneck P, Goetze-Speer B, Schütt-Gerowitt and Speer CP. Inflammatory pulmonary response following colonization of the airways with Ureaplasma urealyticum in preterm infants at risk for bronchopulmonary dysplasia. Presented at the *9th International Workshop on Surfactant Replacement*, May 1994, Israel.

57. Naessens A, Foulon W, Breynaert J and Lauwers S. Serotypes of *Ureaplasma urealyticum* isolated from normal pregnant women and patients with pregnancy complications. *J Clin Microbiol* 1988;**26**:319–322.

58. Crouse DT, Cassell GH, Waites KB, Foster JM and Cassady G. Hyperoxia potentiates *Ureaplasma urealyticum* pneumonia in newborn mice. *Infect Immun* 1990;**58**:3487–3493.

59. Parker RF, Davis JK, Cassell GH et al. Short-term exposure to nitrogen dioxide enhances susceptibility to murine respiratory mycoplasmosis and decreases intrapulmonary killing of *Mycoplasma pulmonis*. *Am Rev Respir Dis* 1989;**140**:502–512.

60. Greenberg DN, Howell RG II, Hensley DM, Jackson CB, Gress M and Del Vecchio VG. Hyperoxia and *Ureaplasma urealyticum* infection in premature rabbits. *Pediatr Res* 1994;**35(part 2)**:297 (abstract).

61. Blanchard A, Hentschel J, Duffy L, Baldus K and Cassell GH. Detection of *Ureaplasma urealyticum* by polymerase chain reaction in the urogenital tract of adults, in amniotic fluid, and in the respiratory tract of newborns. *Clin Infect Dis* 1993;**17(suppl.)**:S148–153.

62. Blanchard A, Yáñez A, Dybvig K, Watson HL, Griffiths G and Cassell GH. Evaluation of intraspecies genetic variation within 16S rRNA gene of *Mycoplasma hominis* and detection by polymerase chain reaction. *J Clin Microbiol* 1993;**31**:1358–1361.

63. Waites KB, Crouse DT and Cassell GH. Antibiotic susceptibilities and therapeutic options for *Ureaplasma urealyticum* infections in neonates. *Pediatr Infect Dis J* 1992;**11**:23–29.

64. Evans RT and Taylor-Robinson D. The incidence of tetracycline-resistant strains of *Ureaplasma urealyticum*. *J Antimicrob Chemother* 1978;**4**:57–63.

65. Palu G, Valisena S, Barile MF and Meloni GA. Mechanisms of macrolide resistance in *Ureaplasma urealyticum*: a study on collection and clinical strains. *Eur J Epidemiol* 1989;**5**:146–153.

66. Waites KB, Sims PJ, Crouse DT et al. Serum concentrations of erythromycin after intravenous infusion in preterm neonates treated for *Ureaplasma urealyticum* infection. *Pediatr Infect Dis J* 1994;**13**:287–293.

67. Waites KB, Cassell GH, Canupp KC and Fernandes PB. In vitro susceptibilities of mycoplasmas and ureaplasmas to the new macrolides and arylfluroquinolones. *Antimicrob Agents Chemother* 1988;**32**:1500–1502.

68. Ichikawa Y, Ninomiya H, Koga H et al. Erythromycin reduces neutrophil and neutrophil-derived elastolytic-like activity in the lower respiratory tract of bronchiolitis patients. *Am Rev Respir Dis* 1992;**146**:196–203.

69. Oisha K, Sonoda F, Kobayashi S et al. Role of interleukin-8 (IL-8) and an inhibitory effect of erythromycin on IL-8 release in the airways of patients with chronic airways diseases. *Infect Immun* 1994;**62**:4145–4152.

70. Burns L and Hodgman J. Studies of prematures given erythromycin estolate. *Am J Dis Child* 1963;**106**:280–288.

71. McCracken GH, Ginsburg CM and Clahsen TML. Pharmacologic evaluation of orally administered antibiotics in infants and children: effect of feeding on bioavailability. *Pediatrics* 1978;**62**:738–743.

72. Crouse DT, Waites KB, Geerts MH, Hamrick WB, Ford JE and Cassell GH. Parenteral erythromycin is not associated with hearing loss in preterm infants. *Clin Res* 1991;**39**:832 (abstract).

73. Gribble MJ and Chow AW. Erythromycin. *Med Clin North Am* 1982;**66**:79–89.

2

Synchronous Intermittent Mandatory Ventilation

Anne Greenough

INTRODUCTION

Few neonates receive neuromuscular blocking agents whilst being ventilated and their respiratory efforts have an important impact on the outcome of mechanical ventilation[1]. If positive pressure inflation and spontaneous inspiration coincide (synchrony), then oxygenation improves[2] and pneumothorax is less likely. Although synchrony can be encouraged during conventional mechanical ventilation (CMV) by shortening inflation time and/or increasing ventilator rate to mimic more closely the premature infant's respiratory pattern[3,4], these manipulations are not always successful[5]. An ideal solution would be to trigger each positive pressure inflation by the infant's inspiratory effort: recent developments in neonatal ventilators have made 'triggered ventilation' possible.

TRIGGERED VENTILATION MODES

In neonatal practice, synchronized intermittent mandatory ventilation (SIMV), like patient triggered ventilation (PTV), is a pressure assist mode in which the patient's inspiratory demand results in a controlled positive pressure inflation. Inspiratory efforts trigger an inflation after an epoch of time following the previous mechanical breath. In SIMV the maximum number of breaths that is supported is controlled by the SIMV preset rate. Thus, if the infant breathes at a rate of 80 breaths per minute (bpm) and the SIMV rate is 30 bpm, the maximum number of supported breaths is 30 and the assisted breaths are interspersed by non-assisted breaths. In contrast, in PTV every breath made by the infant, providing it is of sufficient magnitude to exceed the critical trigger level, will be supported by a positive pressure inflation. Certain ventilators that trigger on every patient breath call this mode assist control (A/C). Here, the delivered rate during PTV can only indirectly be reduced by increasing inflation time, so stimulating the Hering–Breuer reflex and decreasing respiratory rate[6]. In both modes there is a back-up rate: the frequency at which the infant will be ventilated if he or she becomes apnoeic. In SIMV, the 'back-up' rate is the SIMV rate, whereas in PTV it is usually the rate set on CMV immediately before transfer to PTV.

In adult ventilation, SIMV can be a volume assist mode which may be coupled to pressure support ventilation (PSV). During PSV, a constant preset positive airway pressure is maintained during each spontaneous inspiration[7]. PSV has been shown to reduce the work imposed on the respiratory muscles[8]. PSV can be used to reduce or completely remove the work of breathing, which includes the imposed work by the artificial airway and ventilator circuit[9,10]. In adult practice, comparison of SIMV with and without pressure support demonstrated that the addition of pressure support reduced oxygen consumption[11] and shortened the duration of weaning[7].

A further 'trigger' mode is proportional assisted ventilation (PAV), during which the inspiratory flow generated by the patient is amplified by airway pressure applied throughout inspiration. Unlike SIMV or PTV, in this mode the magnitude of ventilatory assistance is varied and is proportional to the patient's effort throughout the respiratory cycle. In addition to the positive pressure delivered during inspiration, a negative pressure, again in proportion to the flow, is delivered in expiration. During PAV, the compliance and resistance of the respiratory system is measured by the ventilator and from those results the amount of ventilatory assistance required to normalize the mechanics of breathing is calculated. This relieves the patient's feelings of dyspnoea. To date, such a system with a pneumatic pressure regulator has been used in rabbits to reduce the resistive workload of breathing[12]. A prototype machine which incorporates PAV in addition to pressure and volume cycled ventilation, SIMV and high frequency ventilation has been produced for use in neonates.

COMPARISON OF TRIGGERING MECHANISMS

During both SIMV and PTV, the infant's respiratory efforts are detected by a triggering device, which, under certain circumstances, then inputs into the ventilator to cause a positive pressure inflation to be delivered to the infant. One condition that must be fulfilled is that the infant's respiratory efforts are of sufficient magnitude to exceed the critical trigger level. That level is dependent on the method of detection of the respiratory efforts and the device's sensitivity. For example, the SLE 2000 (Specialized Laboratory Equipment Ltd) is triggered by a change in airway pressure of greater than or equal to 0.5 cmH$_2$O[13].

A variety of methods have been used to detect the infant's efforts and some have been developed commercially (Table 2.1). The first PTV system which was specifically designed for neonates was the SLE 250 (Specialized Laboratory Equipment Ltd) ventilator with the Graseby MR10 respiration monitor (Specialized Laboratory Equipment Ltd). The monitor detects the infant's respiratory efforts by use of a pressure capsule, which is usually taped to the infant's abdomen. As the infant inspires, the diaphragm descends, causing the abdomen to expand and this signal is then detected by the capsule. In a small series of infants[14] oxygenation and carbon dioxide elimination improved on the PTV system rather than CMV. Unfortunately, the Graseby MR10 monitor has an internal leak that causes progressive damping of the signal: this results in increasing response times and failure rates[19]. In addition, physiological studies, which compared the Graseby MR10 respiration monitor with an airway pressure trigger-

Table 2.1 Patient triggered ventilation and triggering devices

Ventilator	Triggering system
SLE 250	MR10 respiration monitor including Graseby capsule[14]
	Oesophageal balloon[15]
	Pneumotachograph[16]
	Airway pressure T piece[17]
Sechrist IV	Graseby capsule[18]
	Impedance[19,20] Hewlett Packard cardiorespiratory monitor (SAVI)
Infant Star	Graseby capsule[18] (Star Sync)
Bear Cub	Airflow (NVM-1 monitor)[18]
SLE 2000	Airway pressure[18]
Draeger	Airflow[21,22]
Bird VIP	Tidal volume (partner monitor)[19]

ing system in both acute[23] and chronic lung disease[24], demonstrated the airway pressure trigger to be superior. Other triggering devices used with the SLE 250 ventilator included an oesophageal balloon to detect oesophageal pressure changes[15] and a pneumotachograph to detect airflow changes[16]. The former system was not appropriate for long term use as its presence in the oesophagus stimulated increased peristaltic activity[25] and the additional dead space in the airway caused by the latter device was a concern for chronic ventilation. Those triggering systems[15,16] were followed by an airway pressure trigger. This consisted of a very sensitive pressure transducer connected via a T piece sited close to the endotracheal tube. Despite the superior performance of the airway pressure triggering system[23,24], when used with the SLE 250 ventilator to provide long term support, PTV frequently failed in infants ventilated beyond the first week of life[26] or in the first 24 hours[17,27]. The likely explanation for these problems was the relatively long trigger delay. All the above systems employed the electronic circuitry of the MR10 respiration monitor and, when this was abandoned and an airway pressure trigger or a Graseby capsule system with different electronics was used, much shorter trigger delays were experienced[18]. Our own experience, however, indicates that triggered ventilation can be unsuccessful in very immature infants and this relates to the nature of their respiratory efforts[28].

Recent ventilators have used different triggering systems. Although the SLE 2000 has an airway pressure trigger, the ventilator incorporates a resistor in the inspiratory limb of the patient circuit to allow the triggering system to function more sensitively in small infants. Other advantages have been demonstrated for this machine; in particular there is a low volume of compressible gas within the circuit, which improves its efficiency[13,29]. In addition, it produces positive end expiratory pressure (PEEP) and peak inflation pressure (PIP) by separate Venturi flow rates, rather than an exhalation valve, which makes it less prone to inadvertent PEEP at fast rates[30]. Modified transthoracic impedance has also been used as a triggering system[20]. This was originally developed with the Hewlett Packard cardiorespiratory monitor, but the Sechrist interface (SAVI – synchronized assisted ventilation of infants) has now been modified and can be used with other monitors. Flow signals can be detected using thermistors or hot wire anemometers; the use of such devices with one hidden by a baffle allows the direction of gas flow to be detected. A wire mesh screen (pneumotachograph) can also be used (Bear Cub Enhancement Module, CEM). Flow systems have the advantage that tidal and minute volume can be derived from the signal and can be displayed by the ventilator. The disadvantages of the flow sensor systems are added dead space in the airway (approximately 1 ml) and the imposition of an additional resistance load. The Bear CEM, when used for very low birthweight infants, has been associated with carbon dioxide retention[19] and in a laboratory based study was found to have the highest rate of autotriggering of three flow triggered ventilators (Draeger Babylog 8000, Bear Cub CEM, Bird VIP)[31].

It is possible to compare the performance of the different triggering devices by assessing their sensitivity and the ventilator device's speed of response, or the 'trigger delay'. The sensitivity is calculated as the proportion of the infant's efforts that is detected. The response time/trigger delay is the time from the initiation of the infant's respiratory effort to the commencement of the triggered positive pressure inflation. Both the sensitivity and the trigger delay can be measured by simultaneously recording changes in airway pressure and an independent method of recording the infant's respiratory efforts, for example using an oesophageal balloon or diaphragmatic electromyographic signal. A number of comparative studies of ventilators and their triggering devices have been performed[18,31–33]. Clinical studies[18] suggest that the currently available systems perform well, in the majority of premature infants, regardless of whether they have acute or chronic respiratory distress, with trigger delays of less than 150 ms. This cutoff is important, for if triggered ventilation is to provide successful long term support for an infant, then inflation must be delivered in the first half of inspiration[17]. Several studies have documented the inspiratory time of ventilated infants to be between 0.31[34] and 0.35 seconds[35,36]. Thus, if inflation is to be initiated in the first half of inspiration, then the trigger delay must be less than 150 ms. Current evidence suggests that the airway pressure[18] and Graseby capsule[31] triggering systems perform better than airflow systems, but the latter better than an impedance device[32]. For example, in ten preterm neonates the mean response time of the Draeger Babylog 8000 (airflow system) was found to be 111 ms, compared with 167 ms with the SAVI system (impedance device). A further advantage of the airflow triggering system was the absence of autotriggered breaths, whereas with the SAVI system 12.9% of the mechanical breaths were autotriggered[32].

PHYSIOLOGICAL STUDIES

During intermittent mandatory ventilation (IMV), positive pressure inflations are delivered regularly but regardless of the timing of the infant's respiratory efforts. As a consequence, the delivered volume associated with a positive pressure inflation during IMV is variable (Figure 2.1). In SIMV, the patient's respiratory efforts trigger a maximum preset number of ventilator breaths. As the timing of the ventilator breaths is determined by the infant's respiratory efforts, this can be variable (Figure 2.1), but as inflation and inspiration usually coincide, the delivered volume associated with a ventilator breath is greater during SIMV than IMV. In PTV, a ventilator breath is triggered by each and all of the infant's respiratory efforts providing they are of sufficient magnitude to exceed the critical trigger level. As a consequence, during PTV there will be a greater number of supported breaths compared with IMV or SIMV. Inflation and inspiration should coincide in PTV, as in SIMV; thus the delivered volume will be greater in PTV than in IMV (Figure 2.1).

Comparison of short periods of SIMV with CMV have revealed improvements in both tidal volume and blood gases[37]. In 30 infants with respiratory failure the mean tidal volume during SIMV was $7.2 \, \text{ml kg}^{-1}$ compared with $6.2 \, \text{ml kg}^{-1}$ during CMV ($P < 0.01$). A greater variability in tidal volume was found during CMV, and both this and the lower tidal volume were explained by the very low rate of synchronous respiration during CMV. Many infants on CMV showed a mixed pattern of respiratory interaction, and tidal volumes were particularly reduced when IMV breaths began in the first half of spontaneous expiration or during the last half of inspiration[38]. In a subsequent study[39] the lower rate of asynchrony (less than 1%) on SIMV compared with the 52% rate experienced on CMV led to superior blood gases. Twenty-six paired comparisons were made of the two ventilation modes and demonstrated a mean PaO_2 of 61.5 mmHg on SIMV versus 53.3 mmHg on CMV ($P < 0.01$) and a mean $PaCO_2$ of 42.7 mmHg on CMV versus 41.3 mmHg on SIMV ($P < 0.05$)[39].

Hummler et al showed that SIMV reduced blood pressure fluctuations when compared with IMV[40]. Such variations have been implicated as a risk factor in the pathogenesis of intracranial haemorrhage. In a crossover design study[40], using the Draeger ventilator, the significantly higher volume delivery during SIMV compared to IMV was confirmed[37]. In addition, the mean beat to beat variation of both systolic and diastolic blood presssure were lower in the SIMV mode. Regression analysis revealed a significant correlation between peak oesophageal pressure changes and beat to beat blood pressure variations, indicating that the latter were mainly secondary to pleural pressure changes and produced by spontaneous respiration. In support of

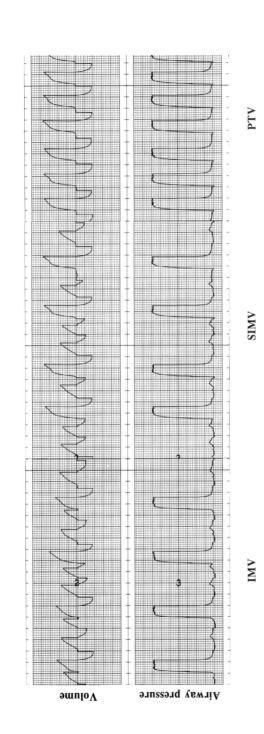

Figure 2.1 Comparison of delivered volume during IMV, SIMV and PTV. The same PIP, PEEP and T_I are used throughout. In addition, the same rate was employed during SIMV and IMV. Lower trace, airway pressure; upper trace, volume: inflation upwards, expiration downwards.

that hypothesis[40], diaphragmatic activity was found to be reduced on SIMV as compared with IMV in healthy animals[41]. The other beneficial effect SIMV has on the cardiovascular system, compared with IMV at identical ventilator settings, is decreased variability in cerebral blood flow velocity[42]. All the above beneficial effects are, as on CMV, likely to occur only if the infant's inspiratory effort and the triggered inflation are synchronous[17] with inflation occurring in the first half of inspiration. Thus the response time/trigger delay of the ventilator triggering device is crucial (see above). Once inflation extends into expiration, this is likely to provoke an active expiratory reflex with reduction in tidal volume and risk of pneumothorax[1]. If the trigger delay is long (>150 ms), the inspiratory time could be shortened to prevent inflation extending into expiration, but below a critical value (0.25 s) delivered volume will be impaired[43].

CLINICAL STUDIES

Acute Respiratory Distress

The advantages of SIMV demonstrated in physiological studies[37,39,40,42] may be translated into clinical gains. In a multicentre trial[44], 306 infants were randomized at a mean age of 7.5 hours to SIMV or IMV. The Infant Star ventilator was used throughout the study and SIMV was delivered by the Star Sync module. The infants had similar birthweight, gestational age, Apgar scores and arterial : alveolar oxygen ratio at the time of randomization. There was no difference in the mortality or IVH rate and the use of neuromuscular blocking agents was similar in the two groups. In infants of birthweight less than 1.0 kg, however, the proportion of infants who required supplementary oxygen at 35 weeks postconceptional age was lower in the SIMV group (46%), compared with 77% in the IMV group ($P<0.05$). Amongst infants of birthweight greater than 2.0 kg, the duration of ventilation was shorter in the SIMV group (median 72 hours), versus 96 hours in the IMV group ($P<0.05$)[44].

Weaning

In SIMV mode, weaning can be achieved by reducing pressure, rate or a combination of both. This gives much greater flexibility than in patient triggered mode because in that mode every one of the infant's respiratory efforts that exceeds the critical trigger level will be supported by a positive pressure inflation. As a consequence, weaning during PTV can only be brought about by reduction in pressure; nevertheless, that has been found to be superior to conventional weaning[45]. In none of three randomized trials[46,47] that recruited premature infants (gestational age <35 weeks) was any advantage shown in terms of shortening the duration of weaning or reducing the need for reintubation associated with SIMV compared with PTV. In all three trials[46,47] infants followed a routine weaning policy[48] until a ventilator rate of 40 bpm was reached, when aminophylline or theophylline was started at 4 mg kg^{-1} day^{-1}. Infants were then randomized to either PTV or SIMV using the SLE 2000 ventilator. The trigger sensitivity was set to maximum, that is, a change in airway pressure within the ventilator circuit of 0.5 cmH$_2$O or greater triggered the ventilator[13]. Weaning during PTV by reduction in pressure was in steps of 2 cmH$_2$O. In the first trial[46], weaning in SIMV mode was by reduction in rate only; inspiratory time and PIP were kept constant; rate reduction was in steps of 5 bpm. In the second trial[47], during SIMV pressure was reduced in 2 cmH$_2$O increments as in PTV, but in addition rate was reduced in steps of 5 bpm, keeping the inspiratory time constant, until a rate of 20 bpm was achieved, whereupon the infant was switched to endotracheal continuous positive airways pressure (CPAP). In the third study[47], in SIMV mode pressure and rate were reduced, but rate was decreased to 5 bpm before switching to CPAP. In all other respects the protocol for weaning was similar for both ventilator modes, and the clinical characteristics of the patients who received SIMV or PTV were not significantly different.

In none of the trials was there any significant difference between modes regarding the number of infants in whom weaning failed (Table 2.2), that is, either no reduction in ventilatory requirements could be made within a 24 hour period or the infant required reintubation within the first 48 hours after extubation. In the first trial, seven of the 12 infants in whom weaning failed were below 27 weeks of gestational age. In the second and third trials, although there was no significant difference in the severity of initial respiratory illness (as evidenced by the maximum inspired oxygen concentration and peak pressure or use of surfactant replacement therapy) between infants in whom weaning failed or succeeded, the former group were more immature (gestational age 26 versus 28 weeks) and of lower birthweight (911 versus 1103 g). These data suggest that currently used indicators of readiness to wean are not universally applicable to extremely low birthweight infants.

Only in the third trial was there a significant difference in the dura-

Table 2.2 Comparison of weaning by SIMV and PTV

	SIMV	PTV	P
Trial 1 (n = 40)[46]			
Weaning failure	6	6	
Duration (hours)	36 (8–647)	22 (4–339)	NS
Trial 2 (n = 40)[47]			
Weaning failure	5	6	
Duration (hours)	30 (7–408)	33 (4–912)	NS
Trial 3 (n = 40)[47]			
Weaning failure	5	2	
Duration (hours)	50 (12–500)	24 (7–432)	<0.05

Data are expressed as the number or median (range).
NS, not significant.

tion of weaning between the ventilator modes, and this favoured PTV (Table 2.2). In SIMV, when rate is reduced this decreases the number of the infant's breaths that are supported by positive pressure. This means that for increasingly longer periods the infant breathes on CPAP through the resistance of the endotracheal tube. This is likely to increase the work of breathing, which would have a negative effect on weaning and hence explain the longer duration of weaning experienced on SIMV, seen particularly in trial three. The data from the trials[46,47] also suggest that there may be a critical number of the infant's breaths that must be supported during weaning from mechanical ventilation. As a significant difference in the duration of weaning was noted only in trial three, this would infer that 20 bpm may be the critical number. The data from all three trials fail to support the concept that, despite the greater flexibility that weaning by SIMV offers, this mode has any advantage over PTV for weaning premature infants.

CONCLUSION

The addition of SIMV mode to currently available neonatal ventilators has increased the flexibility of respiratory support. Evidence to date, however, suggests it does not have a useful role in weaning premature infants ventilated in the first 2 weeks of life. Its niche may be for the term infant whose respiratory efforts are so vigorous that during PTV there would be difficulty in maintaining carbon dioxide tensions – anecdotally we have certainly employed it successfully for such a purpose. The future of SIMV, wherever it may lie, must incorporate proportional assist ventilation.

REFERENCES

1. Greenough A. Pancuronium administration and immediate hypoventilation. *J Pediatr* 1984;**105**:849.
2. Greenough A, Pool J, Greenall F, Morley CJ and Gamsu H. Comparison of different rates of artificial ventilation in preterm neonates with the respiratory distress syndrome. *Acta Paediatr Scand* 1987;**76**:706–712.
3. Greenough A, Greenall F and Gamsu H. Synchronous respiration – which ventilator rate is best? *Acta Paediatr Scand* 1987;**76**:713–718.
4. Field D, Milner AD and Hopkin IE. Manipulation of ventilator settings to reduce expiration against positive pressure inflation. *Arch Dis Child* 1985;**60**:1036–1040.
5. Greenough A, Morley CJ and Pool J. Fighting the ventilator – are fast rates an effective alternative to paralysis? *Early Hum Dev* 1986;**13**:189–194.
6. Upton CJ, Milner AD and Stokes GM. The effect of changes in inspiratory time on neonatal triggered ventilation. *Eur J Pediatr* 1990;**149**:648–650.
7. Jaunieaux V, Duran A and Levi-Valensi P. Synchronized intermittent mandatory ventilation with and without pressure support ventilation in weaning patients with COPD from mechanical ventilation. *Chest* 1994;**105**:1204–1210.
8. Brochard L, Harf A, Lovino H and Leyaire F. Inspiratory pressure support prevents diaphragmatic fatigue during weaning from mechanical ventilation. *Am Rev Respir Dis* 1989;**139**:513–521.
9. Kacmarek RM. The role of pressure support in reducing the work of breathing. *Respir Care* 1988;**33**:99.
10. Fiastro JF, Habib MP and Quan SF. Pressure support compensation for inspiratory work due to endotracheal tubes and demand continuous positive airway pressure. *Chest* 1988;**92**:499–505.
11. Kanak R, Fahey PJ and Vanderwarf C. Oxygen cost of breathing changes dependent upon mode of mechanical ventilation. *Chest* 1985;**87**:126–127.
12. Schulze A, Schaller P, Gerhardt B, Midler H and Gruyrek D. An infant ventilatory technique for resistive unloading during spontaneous breathing. Results in a rabbit model of airway obstruction. *Pediatr Res* 1990;**28**:79–82.
13. Greenough A, Hird MF and Chan V. Airway pressure triggered ventilation for preterm neonates. *J Perinat Med* 1991;**19**:471–476.
14. Mehta A, Callan K, Wright BM and Stacey TE. Patient triggered ventilation in the newborn. *Lancet* 1986;**ii**:17–19.
15. Greenough A and Greenall F. Patient triggered ventilation in premature neonates. *Arch Dis Child* 1988;**63**:77–78.
16. Greenough A and Pool J. Neonatal patient triggered ventilation. *Arch Dis Child* 1988;**63**:394–397.

17. Hird MF and Greenough A. Causes of failure of neonatal patient triggered ventilation. *Early Hum Dev* 1990;**23:**101–108.

18. Chan V and Greenough A. Neonatal patient triggered ventilators. Performance in acute and chronic lung disease. *Br J Intensive Care* 1993;**3:**216–219.

19. Heldt GP and Bernstein G. Patient-initiated mechanical ventilation. In: Boynton BR, Carlo WA and Jobe AH (eds) *New therapies for neonatal respiratory failure. A physiological approach.* Cambridge: Cambridge University Press, 1994: 152.

20. Vishveshwara N, Freeman B, Peck M, Caliwag N, Shook S and Rajani KB. Patient triggered synchronized assisted ventilation of newborns: report of a preliminary study and three years' experience. *J Perinatol* 1991; **11:**347–354.

21. Hird MF and Greenough A. Gestational age: an important influence on the success of patient triggered ventilation. *Clin Phys Physiol Meas* 1990; **11:**307–312.

22. Hird MF and Greenough A. Patient triggered ventilation using a flow triggered system. *Arch Dis Child* 1991;**66:**1140–1143.

23. Hird MF and Greenough A. Comparison of triggering systems for neonatal patient triggered ventilation. *Arch Dis Child* 1991;**66:**426–428.

24. Chan V and Greenough A. Evaluation of triggering systems for patient triggered ventilation for neonates ventilator-dependent beyond 10 days of age. *Eur J Pediatr* 1992;**151:**842–845.

25. Greenough A and Milner AD. Respiratory support using patient triggered ventilation in the neonatal period. *Arch Dis Child* 1991;**67:**69–71.

26. Hird MF and Greenough A. Patient triggered ventilation in chronically ventilator-dependent infants. *Eur J Pediatr* 1991;**150:**732–734.

27. Hird MF and Greenough A. Randomised trial of patient triggered ventilation versus high frequency positive pressure ventilation in acute respiratory distress. *J Perinat Med* 1991;**19:**379–384.

28. Chan V, Greenough A and Muramatsu K. Influence of lung function and reflex activity on the success of patient triggered ventilation. *Early Hum Dev* 1994;**37:**9–14.

29. Chan KN, Chakrabarti MK, Whitwam JG and Silverman M. Assessment of a new valveless infant ventilator. *Arch Dis Child* 1988;**63:**162–167.

30. Chan V, Greenough A and Milner AD. The performance of a new valveless ventilator at rates of up to 250 bpm. *J Perinat Med* 1994;**22:**387–391.

31. Bernstein G, Clearly JP, Heldt GP, Rosas FR, Shellemberg LD and Mannino FL. Response time and reliability of three neonatal patient triggered ventilators. *Am Rev Respir Dis* 1993;**148:**358–364.

32. Hummler H, Gerhardt T, Claure N, Everett R and Bancalari E. Patient triggered ventilation (PTV) in neonates: comparison of an airflow and an impedance triggered system. *Pediatr Res* 1994;**35:**337 (abstract).

33. John L, Bjorklund L, Svenningsen NW and Johnson B. Airway and body surface sensors for triggering in neonatal ventilation. *Acta Paediatr Scand* 1994;**93:**903–909.

34. South M and Morley CJ. Respiratory timing in intubated neonates with respiratory distress syndrome. *Arch Dis Child* 1992;**67**:446–448.

35. Sequin JH, Donovan EF and Kotagal HR. Respiratory timing in newborns with respiratory distress syndrome. *Pediatr Res* 1985;**19**:1515 (abstract).

36. Hird MF and Greenough A. Inflation time in mechanical ventilation of preterm neonates. *Eur J Pediatr* 1991;**150**:440–443.

37. Bernstein G, Heldt GP and Mannino FL. Increased and more consistent tidal volumes during synchronized intermittent mandatory ventilation in newborn infants. *Am J Respir Crit Care* 1994;**150**:1444–1448.

38. Greenough A. The premature infant's respiratory response to mechanical ventilation. *Early Hum Dev* 1988;**17**:1–5.

39. Cleary JP, Bernstein G, Mannino FL and Heldt GP. Improved oxygenation during synchronized intermittent mandatory ventilation in neonates with respiratory distress syndrome: a randomized crossover study. *J Pediatr* 1995;**126**:407–411.

40. Hummler H, Gerhardt T, Claure N, Everett R and Bancalari E. Influence of patient triggered ventilation (PTV) on ventilation and blood pressure fluctuations in neonates. *Pediatr Res* 1994;**35**:338 (abstract).

41. Rosas FR, Clearly JP, Mannino FL, Bernstein G and Heldt GP. Diaphragmatic effort and lung mechanics on conventional ventilation and synchronized intermittent mandatory ventilation (IMV/SIMV). *Pediatr Res* 1992;**32**:148 (abstract).

42. Govindaswami B, Heldt GP, Bernstein G and Bejar R. Reduction in cerebral blood flow velocity (CBFV) variability in infants <1500 g during synchronized ventilation (SIMV). *Pediatr Res* 1993;**33**:1258.

43. Field D, Milner AD and Hopkin IE. Inspiratory time and tidal volume during intermittent positive pressure ventilation. *Arch Dis Child* 1985;**60**:259–261.

44. Bernstein G, Mannino FL, Heldt GP et al. Prospective randomized multi-centre trial comparing synchronized and conventional intermittent mandatory ventilation (SIMV vs IMV) in neonates. *Pediatr Res* 1994;**35**:216 (abstract).

45. Chan V and Greenough A. Randomised controlled trial of weaning by patient triggered ventilation or conventional ventilation. *Eur J Pediatr* 1993;**152**:51–54.

46. Chan V and Greenough A. Comparison of weaning by patient triggered ventilation or synchronous mandatory intermittent ventilation. *Acta Paediatr* 1994;**83**:335–337.

47. Dimitriou G, Greenough A, Giffin F and Chan V. Synchronous intermittent mandatory ventilation modes versus patient triggered ventilation during weaning. *Arch Dis Child* 1996;**72**:F188–F190.

48. Greenough A, Pool J and Gamsu H. A randomised controlled trial of two methods of weaning from high frequency positive pressure ventilation. *Arch Dis Child* 1989;**64**:834–838.

3

Near Infrared Spectroscopy

John S. Wyatt

INTRODUCTION

Near infrared spectroscopy (NIRS) has been employed as a research tool to investigate the newborn brain for approximately 10 years. The aim of this chapter is to outline the fundamental strengths and weaknesses of the technique, review the progress that has been made since clinical studies commenced, and discuss the potential contribution to the care of the newborn infant that NIRS is likely to make in the foreseeable future.

PRINCIPLES

The physical principles of optical transmission spectroscopy were developed during the early part of the twentieth century, but in 1977 Frans Jobsis described the use of near infrared light for spectroscopy of biological tissue in vivo[1]. NIRS depends on two fundamental physical properties of biological tissue: (1) the relative transparency of biological tissue to light in the near infrared region of the spectrum; and (2) the existence within tissue of a small number of colour bearing compounds (known as chromophores) that are present in variable concentrations and whose light absorbing properties vary with oxygenation.

Relative Transparency of Biological Tissue

As light passes through tissue its intensity falls (known technically as optical attenuation) due to a combination of absorption and scattering. Visible light (with wavelengths up to 650 nm) is strongly absorbed within tissue by a number of pigments (especially haemoglobin) and, even with very intense light sources, the maximum distance of photon penetration is only about 1 cm. However, the near infrared region of the spectrum (700–1000 nm) represents an optical 'window' allowing the interrogation of larger volumes of tissue. Light absorption is greatly reduced compared with the visible region, and optical attenuation is dominated by light scattering within the tissues. At these wavelengths, photons can penetrate into tissue for distances of 8 cm or more. Using modern light sources and detectors it is therefore possible to detect and measure near infrared light that has transilluminated a substantial proportion of the newborn infant head[2].

Biological Chromophores

Within the neonatal brain there are only three chromophores (light absorbing compounds) which have significant absorption bands in the near infrared region and which are present in variable concentrations. These are oxyhaemoglobin (HbO_2), deoxyhaemoglobin (Hb) and the oxidized form of the copper A moiety (Cu_A) of cytochrome oxidase, the terminal member of the mitochondrial respiratory chain. Any changes in the concentration of these three chromophores will therefore be reflected in the absorption of near infrared photons passing through the tissue. By using near infrared light with at least three different wavelengths it is possible to obtain simultaneous information about all three chromophores, HbO_2, Hb and Cu_A[3]. Although other chromophores are known to be present within biological tissue (water, bilirubin, etc.), it is assumed that their concentration is constant during the period of optical transillumination.

Quantification of NIRS Measurements

In order to obtain quantification of spectroscopy data it is necessary to convert measurements of optical attenuation into data about the concentration of the relevant chromophores. The relationship between optical absorption and chromophore concentration in a highly scattering medium is described by a modification of the Beer–Lambert law[4]:

$$OD = a.c.L.B + G$$

where OD is the optical density, a is the absorption coefficient of the chromophore (mmol^{-1} cm^{-1}), c is concentration (mmol l^{-1}), and L is the distance (cm) between light entry and exit points. B is a dimensionless 'pathlength factor' which accounts for the increase in optical pathlength caused by scattering, and G is a geometrical factor which accounts for loss of photons by scattering out of the line between the source and detector. If L, B and G remain constant, then *changes* in optical density may be converted into *changes* in chromophore concentration using the relationship:

$$\Delta c = \Delta OD/(a.L.B)$$

If a, L and B are known it is possible to convert changes in optical attenuation (measured in optical densities) into changes in chromophore concentration (in mmol l^{-1}). If more than one chromophore is present it is necessary to measure optical density changes simultaneously at several wavelengths. As there are three chromophores within brain tissue (HbO$_2$, Hb, Cu$_A$), it is necessary to make measurements at a minimum of three different wavelengths and employ a previously derived algorithm[3]. If more than three wavelengths are employed, standard curve fitting analysis may be used to increase the accuracy of the calculated concentration changes.

Estimation of Optical Pathlength

Quantification of NIRS measurements requires knowledge of the average pathlength of the photons traversing the tissue. Because of multiple scattering this pathlength is considerably longer than the distance between the sites of light entry and exit. In order to obtain absolute quantification of chromophore concentration it is therefore necessary to obtain B, the pathlength factor. A number of optical techniques are now becoming available to allow this important variable to be measured in the newborn brain.

The first technique involves the use of a pulsed laser and high speed detector to measure the 'time of flight' of an ultrashort pulse of infrared light as it traverses the head[4]. As the speed of light is known, it is possible to obtain the mean optical pathlength that the photons have travelled within the head. In a post-mortem study of six preterm infants using time of flight measurements a mean value for B of

4.4 ± (SD) 0.3 was obtained[5]. A subsequent study in ten term and preterm infants with varying geometrical arrangements of the optodes gave a value of 3.9 ± (SD) 0.6[6]. Values for *B* were relatively constant provided that the distance between the transmitting and receiving fibres was greater than 2.5 cm. Because of the size and complexity of the equipment required to make time of flight measurements, this technique cannot as yet be employed within a neonatal intensive care unit. It is therefore not possible to measure optical pathlength directly in each baby being studied. However, the optical pathlength can be estimated in any individual by measuring the distance (*L*) between the transmitting and receiving optical fibres and multiplying this distance by a mean value for *B*. Thus if the distance between the optical fibres is 5 cm and a value for *B* of 4.4 is assumed, the optical pathlength is estimated to be 22 cm.

Secondly, it is possible to use the infrared absorption of water molecules in the brain to obtain optical pathlength. As the concentration of water within brain tissue is known (to a reasonable degree of accuracy), it can be employed as a calibration compound and hence provide the optical pathlength in each baby[7]. Preliminary data in a newborn infant provided a value for *B* of 4.5 ± (SD) 0.2. This technique has the advantage that continuous measurements can be obtained at the cotside.

Thirdly, if the transmitted infrared light is modulated by a very high frequency signal, the phase shift between the transmitted and received light can be measured in order to obtain both the optical pathlength and concentration information simultaneously[8,9]. Prototype instruments are now becoming available to enable these measurements to be obtained at the cotside, and preliminary data are currently being obtained from the neonatal and infant brain. Preliminary results using these new techniques suggest that there is a significant variation in optical pathlength between different individuals, although the reasons for this variation are not yet understood. It seems clear therefore that, in future, it will be necessary to use NIRS techniques which allow the direct determination of optical pathlength at the cotside if a high level of accuracy is required.

Theoretical Assumptions

Several theoretical assumptions underlie the quantification of NIRS data. Firstly, it is assumed that there are no other chromophores, apart from HbO_2, Hb and Cu_A, which are present in the light path and whose concentration changes during the measurement period.

Secondly, it is assumed that all the chromophores are distributed homogeneously throughout the brain tissue; and, thirdly, that extra-cerebral tissue such as scalp and bone make a negligible contribution to the NIRS signals. In practice the extracerebral compartment prob-ably contributes less than 5% of the total signal in the newborn, although this percentage is known to be significantly greater in the older child and adult.

QUANTIFICATION OF HAEMODYNAMIC VARIABLES

Once the optodes are positioned on the scalp, and values for L and B are provided, it is then possible to convert any observed optical den-sity *changes* into *changes* in the concentrations of the three principal chromophores [HbO_2], [Hb] and [Cu_A]. In addition, changes in the total haemoglobin concentration [Hb_{tot}] are derived from the sum of changes in [HbO_2] and [Hb]. If data about other circulatory variables are collected simultaneously, absolute quantification of several important physiological variables may be obtained, including cere-bral blood flow, cerebral blood volume and its response to changing arterial carbon dioxide tension.

Cerebral Blood Flow

Global cerebral blood flow (CBF) may be obtained by employing a version of the Fick principle which employs oxyhaemoglobin as an endogenous intravascular tracer molecule[10,11]. A pulse oximeter, modified to provide beat to beat measurements, is used to provide a continuous estimate of arterial saturation (SaO_2) and the inspired oxygen concentration is adjusted to give a stable arterial saturation in the region of 85–90%. Following baseline measurements, a rapid transient increase in the inspired oxygen concentration is induced over a few seconds, leading to a rapid increase in SaO_2 of 5–10%. The resultant rise in cerebral [HbO_2] is measured by NIRS. If cerebral perfusion and oxygen extraction remain constant during this proce-dure, global CBF (in ml 100 g^{-1}min^{-1}) can then be obtained[10]. Cerebral oxygen delivery (COD) can also be derived, if the small quantity of oxygen dissolved in plasma is ignored. The fundamental theory underlying this method for determining CBF has been dis-cussed in more detail elsewhere[11]. Two recent studies in newborn infants undergoing intensive care have shown a close correlation between CBF measurements obtained by NIRS and by the intravenous xenon-133 technique[12,13]. In addition to the oxyhaemoglobin method for obtaining CBF, an alternative technique that uses indocyanine green as an exogenous tracer has been recently described in infants undergoing cardiopulmonary bypass[14].

Cerebral Blood Volume

Global cerebral blood volume (CBV) is obtained by observing the effect on cerebral [HbO_2] of a small and gradual change in SaO_2 of 5–10% induced over about 5 minutes by a gradual change of inspired oxygen concentration[15]. If cerebral oxygen extraction can be assumed to remain constant during this manoeuvre, total cerebral haemoglobin concentration (in mmol l^{-1}) may be obtained from the change in [HbO_2], using a modification of a standard indicator dilution technique. The total haemoglobin concentration may then be converted to CBV (in ml 100 g^{-1}), by measuring the blood haemoglobin concentration from a sample taken from a peripheral vein and assuming a value for the cerebral:large vessel haematocrit ratio and for brain density[15].

CBV Response to Changing Arterial Carbon Dioxide Concentration

The response of CBV to changing arterial carbon dioxide concentration (CBVR) (measured in ml 100 g^{-1} kPa^{-1}) may be determined by measuring the change in total cerebral haemoglobin concentration in response to a small gradual change in the arterial carbon dioxide tension ($PaCO_2$)[16,17]. This change may be induced by a small change in ventilator rate, or, in more mature infants who are clinically stable, by adding a small amount of exogenous carbon dioxide to the inspired air. During this manoeuvre the arterial oxygen saturation is maintained as constant as possible. $PaCO_2$ is measured from an arterial blood gas specimen or estimated continuously using a transcutaneous electrode.

Cerebral Venous Oxygen Saturation

An estimate of cerebral venous oxygen saturation may be obtained by investigating the effect of briefly tilting the infant head down[18,19]. If it is assumed that any increase in cerebral blood volume is dominated by changes in the venous compartment then the venous saturation is obtained from the ratio of the change in [HbO_2] compared with [Hb_{tot}].

Advantages and Limitations in the Use of NIRS to Measure Cerebral Haemodynamics

NIRS has obvious advantages as a practical tool for measurement of haemodynamic variables in sick newborn infants. No ionizing radiation is employed, no exogenous tracer need be administered and measurements can be obtained at the cotside. Provided that a suitable small change can be induced in SaO_2, estimations of CBF and CBV may be performed repeatedly without risk and with minimal interference to the infant. However, there are several important limitations in the usefulness of NIRS as a practical clinical measuring device at present. In infants with normal lungs, SaO_2 is frequently above 97% while room air is breathed. Thus it may not be possible to induce a suitable rise in SaO_2 despite the administration of additional oxygen. (It would be possible, in theory, to administer a hypoxic gas mixture in order to cause SaO_2 to fall to around 90% before the administration of additional oxygen, but this approach has not yet been described in the newborn infant.) Conversely, in infants with severe lung disease, or other conditions associated with right to left shunting of blood, SaO_2 may be fixed at a low level, with no significant rise despite administration of pure oxygen. Thus satisfactory measurements of CBF and CBV may not be possible in a significant proportion of infants. For reliable measurements of CBV and CBF no significant change in cerebral perfusion should occur during a small change in SaO_2. However, in some infants, an unpredictable variation in CBV may be observed when SaO_2 changes, leading to a significant inaccuracy in the measurement of haemodynamic variables. Finally, deficiencies in the quality of the pulse oximetry data may also lead to inaccuracies in continuous SaO_2 measurement, leading to errors in the determination of CBF and CBV.

DATA OBTAINED BY NIRS IN NEWBORN INFANTS

Several groups have reported results from studies using NIRS in newborn infants undergoing intensive care. Brazy[20] showed relative changes in [HbO_2], [Hb] and [Cu_A] with crying and nursing procedures. They also reported that spontaneous fluctuations in arterial blood pressure were associated with changes in CBV and [Cu_A][21]. In a study of nine preterm infants with intermittent episodes of apnoea and bradycardia, Livera and colleagues detected sharp falls in [HbO_2] and in CBV[22] and in a study of endotracheal suctioning, Shah and colleagues demonstrated marked transient fluctuations in cerebral oxygenation and perfusion[23]. Absolute quantification of the NIRS data was not possible.

Measurements of Cerebral Blood Volume

Wyatt and colleagues measured CBV in 12 term and preterm infants who were undergoing intensive care but who were thought to have normal brains[15]. Mean CBV was 2.2 ± (SD) 0.4 ml 100 g^{-1}, similar to values obtained by positron emission tomography. In this small group of patients there was no evidence of a systematic change in CBV with increasing gestational age. In a further ten infants who had evidence of brain injury (thought to be mostly hypoxic-ischaemic), mean CBV was significantly elevated at 3.0 ± (SD) 1.0 ml 100 g^{-1}. In another study of 12 term infants with hypoxic-ischaemic encephalopathy following perinatal asphyxia, studied in the first 48 hours after birth, CBV was found to be elevated with a mean value of 4.4 ± (SEM) 0.4 ml 100 g^{-1} compared with a mean value of 2.0 ± (SEM) 0.3 ml 100 g^{-1} in six control infants[24]. In a further study McCormick and colleagues investigated the relationship between early haemodynamic changes and long term outcome in encephalopathic infants following perinatal asphyxia[25]. Twenty-one term infants were studied in the first 24 hours after birth. Eight of 21 infants subsequently died and the remaining infants were assessed at 1 year of age. Of the variables measured, CBV appeared to be the most closely correlated with outcome, with high CBV associated with adverse outcome. Mean CBV was 6.5 ± (SD) 1.2 ml 100 g^{-1} in infants who died, compared with 3.9 ± (SD) 0.9 ml 100 g^{-1} in infants with a good outcome. A novel method for validation of NIRS data has been described in a study by Wickramsinghe and colleagues employing jugular venous plethysmography and simultaneous measurements from the head using NIRS and a conventional mercury strain gauge[26]. A close correlation between the two methods was obtained.

Measurements of Cerebral Blood Flow

Edwards and coworkers first obtained measurements of CBF in a heterogeneous group of infants undergoing intensive care[10], using oxyhaemoglobin as an intravascular tracer. A mean value of 18 ml 100 g^{-1} min^{-1} was obtained in 13 infants. Subsequently Skov et al[12] and Bucher et al[13] demonstrated a close correlation between simultaneously acquired measurements of CBF by NIRS and by the intravenous xenon-133 technique. Edwards and colleagues demonstrated a marked reduction in CBF and CBV in very preterm infants following administration of indomethacin for closure of a patent ductus arteriosus[27], whereas only minimal changes were observed following surfactant administration[28]. McDonnell and colleagues used similar techniques to demonstrate a significant reduction in CBF following intravenous aminophylline infusion[29].

Measurements of the Cerebrovascular Response to Carbon Dioxide

Several groups have investigated the physiological response of vasodilatation of the cerebral vasculature in response to changing arterial carbon dioxide tension[16,17]. Measurements of the response of CBV to an induced change in carbon dioxide tension (CBVR) gave values that ranged from 0.1 to 0.7 ml 100 g^{-1} kPa^{-1} in 14 term and preterm infants undergoing intensive care[16]. A close linear correlation between CBVR and gestational age was observed, with a marked increase in the cerebrovascular response to changing $PaCO_2$ with increasing maturity. Attenuation of CBVR has been observed in encephalopathic infants following perinatal asphyxia[24,25], indicating disruption of normal vascular control mechanisms. Brun and Greisen have recently published a study of the effects of changing arterial carbon dioxide tension on CBV in 15 preterm infants, indicating discrepancies between measurements obtained from the change in [Hb$_{tot}$] and those from employing the oxygen method to determine CBV[30]. The reasons underlying these discrepancies are not clear, although the authors suggested that changes in the scattering properties of the brain with changing CBV might be responsible. Further fundamental studies on the nature of absorption and scattering changes within the brain are required to clarify this issue.

Measurements of Cerebral Venous Saturation

Although very few data have been published on cerebral venous saturation measured by NIRS, Skov and colleagues[19] showed that venous saturation was significantly elevated in encephalopathic term infants compared with controls, indicating reduced cerebral oxygen extraction probably due to a combination of cerebrovascular vasodilatation and impaired cerebral oxygen consumption following hypoxic-ischaemic brain injury.

Measurements of the Redox State of Cytochrome Oxidase

The fact that cytochrome oxidase displays an absorption peak within the near infrared region has strengthened the potential value of NIRS because it offers the possibility that previously inaccessible information on intracellular oxygen metabolism could be obtained by a non-invasive optical method[1,3,31]. Although several workers have published data on changes in $[Cu_A]$ observed in newborn infants[21,32,33], questions still remain about the possibility of cross-talk with the haemoglobin signals and the correct interpretation of changes in the Cu_A redox state[31]. Skov and Greisen showed that the use of a conventional algorithm led to an overestimate of the real changes in $[Cu_A]$ during induction of cardiopulmonary bypass[34] but the use of a new algorithm with wavelength specific pathlength factors[35] appeared to give more accurate results. Studies comparing the performance of different measurement algorithms in providing accurate Cu_A data have been performed[36] and further work is urgently required to clarify the unresolved issues.

MEASUREMENTS FROM THE FETAL BRAIN DURING LABOUR

The role of NIRS has recently been extended to the fetus during labour[37,38]. Using a specially designed flexible optical probe, which is inserted through the cervix and positioned on the fetal scalp, it is possible to obtain continuous measurements from the fetal brain during labour. The rubber moulding ensures that the sites of light entry and exit are maintained at a constant and known separation from one another. This minimizes the possibility of artefact due to changes in the distance between the optodes. The moulding also ensures that apposition of the optodes to the fetal scalp is maintained throughout the monitoring process. It is shaped like a suction cup and is held in position by the continuous application of mild negative pressure, aided by pressure from the surrounding maternal tissues. Once the cervix is dilated by 2 cm the probe is easily applied to the fetal scalp, after rupture of the amniotic membranes, by introducing it between the fetal head and cervix. Observations may be continued throughout labour and, where feasible, until the point of delivery and beyond[37].

Effect of Uterine Contractions

Large fluctuations in $[HbO_2]$ and $[Hb]$ are routinely observed during each uterine contraction as a result of changes in CBV as the fetal head is mechanically compressed against the maternal perineum. In one preliminary study[37] both [HbO$_2$] and [Hb] fell by a mean of 0.50 ± (SD) 0.27 µmol 100 g^{-1} brain tissue and 0.78 ± (SD) 0.60 µmol 100 g^{-1} respectively. Total haemoglobin concentration ([HbO$_2$] + [Hb]) fell by 1.15 ± (SD) 0.60 µmol 100 g^{-1}, equivalent to a fall in cerebral blood volume of 0.70 ± (SD) 0.39 ml 100 g^{-1}.

Calculation of Mean Cerebral Oxygen Saturation

When both [HbO$_2$] and [Hb] change in the same direction during a contraction, it is possible to calculate the mean cerebral oxygen saturation (SmcO$_2$) from the ratio between the changes in [HbO$_2$] and [Hb$_{tot}$][37,39].

$$SmcO_2 = (100 \times \Delta[HbO_2]) / \Delta([HbO_2]+[Hb])$$

For example, it can be seen that if the changes in [HbO$_2$] and [Hb] are equal, the mean saturation of the cerebral blood leaving and entering the head is 50%. To improve the accuracy of estimation of SmcO$_2$ measurements are usually repeated over several contractions and the mean value obtained. The estimation of SmcO$_2$ by NIRS represents an average saturation of blood within the brain and includes a contribution from all vascular compartments, although it is likely that the measurement is dominated by the cerebral venous compartment. A study of SmcO$_2$ in 33 fetuses undergoing labour gave values within a surprisingly wide range of 21–72%[39]. A strong correlation was found between SmcO$_2$ measured within 30 minutes of delivery and measurements of umbilical artery and vein pH immediately after delivery. A further study demonstrated that fetal cerebral oxygenation during labour is influenced by the rapidity of uterine contractions[40], with very rapid contractions leading to a progressive deoxygenation of the fetal brain. Another study investigated the effect of maternal oxygen administration during labour[41]. A small but significant increase in fetal SmcO$_2$ was detected. Recently maternal posture[42] and pushing[43] during the second stage of labour have also been shown to influence fetal cerebral oxygenation, and a clear association between late fetal rate decelerations and a fall in fetal oxygenation after the uterine contraction has been demonstrated[44]. Although studies are still at an early stage, NIRS performed during labour has obvious potential as a research tool for exploring the effects of normal and abnormal labour on fetal cerebral oxygenation, and for investigating the adaptation of the cerebral circulation to labour and delivery.

RECENT DEVELOPMENTS IN NIRS METHODOLOGY

Wide Band Continuous Spectroscopy

Although most studies with NIRS have employed spectrometers with a small number of discrete near infrared wavelengths, it is possible to transilluminate the infant brain using an intense white light source and a wide band spectrometer coupled to a sensitive light detector[45]. This technique has several advantages. Firstly, because data are obtained simultaneously at a large number of wavelengths, curve fitting techniques can be used to reduce measurement errors. Secondly, the optical pathlength can be measured continuously using the absorption peak of water, thus allowing more accurate determination of chromophore concentration changes[7]. Thirdly, by using curve fitting to detect the unique spectral features of the deoxyhaemoglobin spectrum it is possible to obtain continuous absolute quantification of deoxyhaemoglobin concentration without the need to manipulate SaO_2[46]. Preliminary measurements using this technique are promising and suggest that it may extend the accuracy and range of measurements that can be obtained by NIRS in the neonatal brain.

Frequency Resolved Spectroscopy

This new technique employs continuous laser light on which is superimposed very high frequency intensity modulation. By measuring the phase shift between the incident and transmitted light it is possible to obtain continuous optical pathlength information together with measurements of light attenuation[8,9]. Preliminary data using a prototype instrument have been obtained[47], including pilot studies in newborn infants. By providing continuous information on optical scattering in addition to absorption due to chromophores, frequency resolved spectroscopy may eventually enable detection of *functional* changes in brain tissue which are associated with small scattering changes in the activated brain region.

Future Technical Developments in NIRS

This field is developing very rapidly and by the year 2000 it seems likely that new NIRS instruments will be designed that will be capable of providing both detailed *spatial* information about Hb, HbO_2 and Cu_A within the neonatal brain and relatively accurate absolute quantification of chromophore concentrations. This will enable brain oxygenation and perfusion to be assessed within several anatomical regions at the bedside, without the need to induce changes in SaO_2 or carbon dioxide tension. Sophisticated software and considerable computing power will be required to perform complex data analysis and provide clinically relevant information in real time at the cotside.

CONCLUSION

NIRS has enormous potential for providing non-invasive information about cerebral oxygenation and haemodynamics in the newborn infant undergoing intensive care. Near infrared spectrometers that are currently available can provide valuable research information about cerebral haemodynamics but they have a limited role as practical clinical monitors on the intensive care unit. Technical developments are now occurring at a rapid pace and, in future, NIRS is likely to play an important role in neonatology, providing detailed quantitative and regional information about brain oxygenation and perfusion at the cotside in a form accessible to clinicians.

REFERENCES

1. Jobsis FF. Non-invasive infrared monitoring of cerebral and myocardial sufficiency and circulatory parameters. *Science* 1977;**198:**1264–1267.
2. Cope M and Delpy DT. A system for long-term measurement of cerebral blood and tissue oxygenation in newborn infants by near-infrared transillumination. *Med Biol Eng Comput* 1992;**26:**289–294.
3. Wray SC, Cope M, Delpy DT, Wyatt JS and Reynolds EOR. Characterisation of the near infrared absorption spectra of cytochrome aa₃ and haemoglobin for the non-invasive monitoring of cerebral oxygenation. *Biochim Biophys Acta* 1988;**933:**184–192.
4. Delpy DT, Cope M, van der Zee P, Arridge SR, Wray SC and Wyatt JS. Estimation of optical pathlength through tissue by direct time of flight measurement. *Phys Med Biol* 1988;**33:**1433–1442.
5. Wyatt JS, Cope M, Delpy DT et al. Measurement of optical pathlength for cerebral near infrared spectroscopy in newborn infants. *Dev Neurosci* 1990;**12:**140–144.
6. van der Zee P, Cope M, Arridge SR et al. Experimentally measured optical pathlengths for the adult head, calf and forearm and the head of the newborn infant as a function of inter optode spacing. *Adv Exp Med Biol* 1991;**316:**143–153.
7. Matcher SJ, Cope M and Delpy DT. Use of the water absorption spectrum

to quantify tissue chromophore concentration changes in near-infrared spectroscopy. *Phys Med Biol* 1994;**39:**177–196.

8. Lakowicz JR and Berndt K. Frequency domain measurements of photon migration in tissues. *Chem Phys Lett* 1990;**166:**246–252.

9. Duncan A, Whitlock TL, Cope M and Delpy DT. A multiwavelength, wide-band, intensity modulated optical spectrometer for near infrared spectroscopy and imaging. *Proc Society of Photo-optical Instrumentation Engineers* 1993;**1888:**248–257.

10. Edwards AD, Wyatt JS, Richardson C, Delphy DT, Cope M and Reynolds EOR. Cotside measurement of cerebral blood flow in ill newborn infants by near infrared spectroscopy. *Lancet* 1988;**ii:**770–771.

11. Elwell CE, Cope M, Edwards AD, Wyatt JS, Reynolds EOR and Delpy DT. Measurement of cerebral blood flow in adult humans using near infrared spectroscopy – methodology and possible errors. *Adv Exp Med Biol* 1992;**317:**235–245.

12. Skov L, Pryds O and Greisen G. Estimating cerebral blood flow in newborn infants: comparison of near infrared spectroscopy and [133]xenon clearance. *Pediatr Res* 1991;**30:**570–573.

13. Bucher HU, Edwards AD, Lipp AE and Duc G. Comparison between near infrared spectroscopy and xenon clearance for estimation of cerebral blood flow in critically ill preterm infants. *Pediatr Res* 1993;**33:**56–60.

14. Roberts I, Fallon P, Kirkham FJ et al. Estimation of cerebral blood flow with near infrared spectroscopy and indocyanine green. *Lancet* 1993;**342:**1425.

15. Wyatt JS, Cope M, Delpy DT et al. Quantitation of cerebral blood volume in newborn infants by near infrared spectroscopy. *J Appl Physiol* 1990;**68:**1086–1091.

16. Wyatt JS, Edwards AD, Cope M et al. Response of cerebral blood volume to changes in arterial carbon dioxide tension in preterm and term infants. *Pediatr Res* 1991;**29:**553–557.

17. Pryds O, Greisen G, Skov LL and Friis-Hansen B. Carbon dioxide related changes in cerebral blood volume and cerebral blood flow in mechanically ventilated preterm neonates. Comparison of near infrared spectrophotometry and [133] xenon clearance. *Pediatr Res* 1990;**27:**445–449.

18. Wyatt JS, Cope M, Delpy DT, Wray SC and Reynolds EOR. Quantification of cerebral oxygenation and haemodynamics in sick newborn infants by near infrared spectroscopy. *Lancet* 1986;**ii:**1063–1066.

19. Skov L, Pryds O, Greisen G and Lou H. Estimation of cerebral venous saturation in newborn infants by near infrared spectroscopy. *Pediatr Res* 1993;**33:**52–55.

20. Brazy JE. Effects of crying on cerebral blood volume and cytochrome aa3. *J Pediatr* 1988;**112:**457–461.

21. Brazy JE and Lewis DV. Changes in cerebral blood volume and cytochrome aa3 during hypertensive peaks in preterm infants. *J Pediatr* 1986;**108:**983–987.

22. Livera LN, Spencer SA, Thorniley MS, Wickramsinghe YABD and Rolfe P. The effects of hypoxaemia and bradycardia on neonatal cerebral haemodynamics. *Arch Dis Child* 1991;**66:**376–380.

23. Shah AR, Kurth CD and Gwiazdowski SG. Fluctuations in cerebral oxygenation and blood volume during endotracheal suctioning in premature infants. *J Pediatr* 1992;**120:**769–774.

24. Wyatt JS, Edwards AD, Azzopardi D et al. Cerebral haemodynamics during failure of oxidative phosphorylation following birth asphyxia. *Pediatr Res* 1989;**26:**511 (abstract).

25. McCormick DC, Edwards AD, Roth SC et al. Relation between cerebral haemodynamics and outcome in birth asphyxiated infants studied by near infrared spectroscopy. *Pediatr Res* 1994;**30:**637 (abstract).

26. Wickramsinghe YABD, Livera LN, Spencer SA, Rolfe P and Thorniley MS. Plethysmographic validation of near infrared spectroscopic monitoring of cerebral blood volume. *Arch Dis Child* 1992;**67:**407–411.

27. Edwards AD, Wyatt JS, Richardson C et al. Effects of indomethacin on cerebral haemodynamics in very preterm infants. *Lancet* 1991;**335:** 1491–1495.

28. Edwards AD, McCormick DC, Roth SC et al. Cerebral haemodynamic effects of treatment with modified natural surfactant investigated by near infrared spectroscopy. *Pediatr Res* 1992;**32:**532–536.

29. McDonnell M, Ives NK and Hope PL. Intravenous aminophylline and cerebral blood flow in preterm infants. *Arch Dis Child* 1992;**67:**416–418.

30. Brun NC and Greisen G. Cerebrovascular responses to carbon dioxide as detected by near infrared spectrophotometry: comparison of three different measures. *Pediatr Res* 1994;**36:**20–24.

31. Cooper CE, Matcher SJ, Wyatt JS et al. Near infrared spectroscopy of the brain: relevance to cytochrome oxidase bioenergetics. *Biochem Soc Trans* 1994;**22:**974–980.

32. Edwards AD, Brown GC, Cope M et al. Quantification of changes in the concentration of oxidised cerebral cytochrome oxidase. *J Appl Physiol* 1991;**71:**1907–1913.

33. McCormick DC, Edwards AD, Brown GC et al. Effect of indomethacin on cerebral oxidised cytochrome oxidase in preterm infants. *Pediatr Res* 1993;**33:**603–608.

34. Skov L and Greisen G. Apparent cerebral cytochrome aa3 reduction during cardiopulmonary bypass in hypoxaemic children with congenital heart disease. A critical analysis of in vivo near infrared spectrophotometric data. *Physiol Meas* 1994;**15:**447–457.

35. Essenpreis M, Elwell CE, Cope M, van der Zee P, Arridge SR and Delpy DT. Spectral dependence of temporal point spread function in human tissues. *Appl Opt* 1993;**32:**418–425.

36. Matcher SJ, Elwell CE, Cooper CE, Cope M and Delpy DT. Performance comparison of several published tissue near-infrared spectroscopy algorithms. *Anal Biochem* 1995;**227:**54–68.

37. Peebles DM, Edwards AD, Wyatt JS et al. Changes in human fetal cerebral hemoglobin concentration and oxygenation during labour measured by near-infrared spectroscopy. *Am J Obstet Gynecol* 1992;**166:**1369–1373.

38. Faris F, Doyle M, Wickramsinghe YABD, Houston R, Rolfe P and O'Brien

S. A noninvasive optical technique for intrapartum fetal monitoring: preliminary clinical studies. *Med Eng Phys* 1994;**16**:287–291.

39. Aldrich CJ, D'Antona D, Wyatt JS, Spencer JAD, Peebles DM and Reynolds EOR. Fetal cerebral oxygenation measured by near infrared spectroscopy shortly before birth and acid–base status at birth. *Obstet Gynecol* 1994;**84**:861–866.

40. Peebles DM, Spencer JAD, Edwards AD et al. Relation between frequency of uterine contractions and human fetal cerebral oxygen saturation studied during labour by near infrared spectroscopy. *Br J Obstet Gynaecol* 1994;**101**:44–48.

41. Aldrich CJ, Wyatt JS, Spencer JAD, Reynolds EOR and Delpy DT. The effect of maternal oxygen administration on human fetal cerebral oxygenation measured during labour by near infrared spectroscopy. *Br J Obstet Gynaecol* 1994;**101**:509–513.

42. Aldrich CJ, D'Antona D, Spencer JAD et al. The effect of maternal posture on human fetal cerebral oxygenation during labour with epidural anaesthesia measured by near infrared spectroscopy. *Br J Obstet Gynaecol* 1995;**102**:14–19.

43. Aldrich CJ, D'Antona D, Spencer JAD et al. The effect of maternal pushing on fetal cerebral oxygenation and blood volume during the second stage of labour. *Br J Obstet Gynaecol* 1995;**102**:448–453.

44. Aldrich CJ, D'Antona D, Spencer JAD et al. Late fetal heart decelerations and changes in cerebral oxygenation during the first stage of labour. *Br J Obstet Gynaecol* 1995;**102**:9–13.

45. Cope M, Delpy DT, Wyatt JS, Wray SC and Reynolds EOR. A CCD spectrometer to quantitate the concentration of chromophores in living tissue utilising the absorption peak of water at 975 nm. *Adv Exp Med Biol* 1989;**247**:33–41.

46. Matcher SJ and Cooper CE. Absolute quantification of deoxyhaemoglobin concentration in tissue near infrared spectroscopy. *Phys Med Biol* 1994;**39**:1296–1312.

47. Duncan A, Meek JH, Tyszczuk L et al. Optical pathlength measurements on adult head, calf and forearm and the head of the newborn infant using phase resolved optical spectroscopy. *Phys Med Biol* 1995;**40**:1–10.

4

Fluid Management in the Extremely Preterm Infant

Gunnar Sedin

INTRODUCTION

During fetal life there is an exchange of water and electrolytes between the mother and the fetus through the placental circulation. The fetus also contributes to the formation of amniotic fluid with urine[1] and with water, which is transported through the respiratory tract[2,3] or passes through the skin[4].

The content of body water and its composition in the fetus are related to gestational age[5]. In early gestation the body water amounts to more than 90% of the fetal body weight. During gestation the total body water and extracellular water decrease and the contents of sodium and chloride also decrease proportionally. Intracellular water increases towards the end of term gestation. A fullterm newborn infant has a water content of 77% of the body weight[5]. In preterm infants the total body water at birth is even higher than in fullterm infants, namely 82% at 32 weeks of gestation, 84% at 28 weeks and 86% at 24 weeks[5].

This chapter will deal with fluid management in the most preterm infants. Before the question of fluid therapy can be discussed, it is necessary to present the important matters of body water and sensible and insensible fluid losses that occur in the early period after birth.

POSTNATAL CHANGES IN BODY WATER

After birth the total body water and the extracellular water of the infant continue to decrease[5] and there is a decrease in body weight. This is considered to be a 'physiological weight reduction', the magnitude and duration of which are influenced by the supply of water, electrolytes and nutrients. In extremely preterm infants it is difficult to determine what level of weight reduction is physiological, as the feedback mechanisms such as hunger and thirst are poorly developed and the infants have no ability to manage their own intake. Several regulatory systems are immature and the function of others has not been well studied in extremely preterm infants[6-9]. For the maintenance of cellular functions and for the wellbeing of the infant however, it is necessary to maintain a balance between sodium and water homeostasis during the postnatal changes in the body content of water and electrolytes.

In infants born at a gestational age of 26–30 weeks, Bauer and coworkers[10] found that the total body water decreased by 11.5% from birth until the infants had reached their minimal weight. The change in body water consisted of a loss of extracellular and interstitial volume, while the plasma volume and blood volume remained unchanged. When weight gain started, there was a positive fluid balance. The plasma volume did not change. In this study by Bauer and coworkers total fluid loss exceeded fluid intake because of the high extrarenal water loss on day 1 and the increased diuresis on the following days. Sodium balance was negative initially, with losses of 2.6–7.6 mmol kg^{-1} day^{-1}. These losses became much lower when the initial body weight was regained (3.2 mmol kg^{-1} day^{-1}).

POSTNATAL LOSS OF WATER AND ELECTROLYTES

In the extremely preterm infant water is lost from the skin surface, from the respiratory tract and through the urine and stools. Extremely preterm infants have no ability to sweat[11] and their cutaneous losses are insensible. Very preterm infants are probably unable to increase their water loss from the skin in response to thermal or emotional stimuli[11-13]. At least initially no water can be lost through tears in infants whose eyes are still sealed.

Loss of Water and Electrolytes with Urine

This is the most important form of sensible water loss. In preterm infants born at 26–30 weeks of gestation the water lost with the urine can be around 40 ml kg^{-1} during the first day and may increase to 130 ml kg^{-1} a day on the third day after birth[10]. Infants born at 29–34 weeks of gestation[14] can produce a urine volume of 90 ml kg^{-1} a day early after birth and up to 150 ml kg^{-1} a day on the third day after birth.

Very preterm infants that are well hydrated have a natriuresis/diuresis during the first days after birth while the body weight is decreasing. During this period extra administration of sodium should be avoided. If the sodium load is increased, as a consequence of increased protein intake or administration of extra sodium, the limited renal capacity of very low birthweight infants to concentrate their urine will lead to an increasing urine volume and may result in dehydration[7–9,15,16]. The limited capacity to concentrate urine is considered to be due to unresponsiveness to antidiuretic hormone (ADH)[9], probably with physiological rather than inappropriate ADH secretion[17].

Knowledge of how extremely preterm infants regulate their water and electrolyte balance is not extensive. Critically ill preterm infants with lung disorders and with a restricted sodium supply may have an exaggerated stimulus for renin–angiotensin and increased aldosterone release. These observations have not been made in extremely preterm infants[6]. In studies focused on the role of atrial natriuretic factor (ANF) in postnatal changes in the body fluid compartment in preterm infants[18], no causal relationship was found between the plasma level of ANF and the sodium excretion rate 2–5 days after birth. Other investigators observed a gradual maturation in the effects of ANF, indicating a non-renal role over the first 3–4 postnatal days[19]. During this period ANF may influence water balance by increasing endothelial permeability, which may contribute to respiratory distress[20].

Water Loss with the Stools

Information about water loss with the stools in very preterm and extremely preterm infants is very limited. In healthy term newborn infants, approximately 10 ml kg^{-1} day^{-1} of water is considered to be lost with the stools[21]. In very low birthweight infants born at 30.9 ± (SD) 1.6 weeks of gestation, stool water losses of 7 ml kg^{-1} day^{-1} have been found[22], and this water loss increased during the first week postnatally.

Water Loss from the Skin

The passage of water through the skin of very preterm newborn infants might be due to passive diffusion[23]. While term infants have a cornified layer in the epidermis, which can act as a barrier to water transport, very preterm infants have a poorly developed epidermal layer, with only 2–3 cell layers[24], and there is no efficient barrier to diffusion of water. The amount of water that passes through the skin of very preterm infants depends partly on environmental factors such as humidity and temperature[13,25,26,29]. Transepidermal water loss (TEWL) is usually determined in term and preterm infants with a gradient method (the evaporimeter)[25,27], by measuring the evaporation rate (ER; g m^{-2} h^{-1}) from the chest, an interscapular skin area and a buttock[25].

TEWL at birth and at different postnatal ages

During the first day after birth the rate of evaporation from the skin surface is very high[26,28]. There is an exponential relationship between transepidermal water loss and gestational age in appropriate for gestational age (AGA) infants, with up to 15 times higher TEWL values in infants born at 25 weeks of gestation than in fullterm infants[26]. The curve has a very steep course at gestational ages lower than 28 weeks, and the water losses from the skin surface differ markedly between infants born at 25 weeks and those born at 28 weeks of gestation (Figure 4.1).

The relation between TEWL and gestational age at different postnatal ages during the first 4 weeks after birth can be described with exponential equations (Figure 4.1). The difference in TEWL between the most preterm and fullterm infants gradually diminishes with age, but at a postnatal age of 4 weeks TEWL is still twice as high in the former as in the latter. Among the small for gestational age infants (SGA), TEWL is highest in the most preterm infants, but early after birth the water loss from the skin is lower in SGA infants than in AGA infants of corresponding gestational age at birth[13,28].

Shortly after birth the transepidermal water loss decreases rapidly in the very preterm infant. This is illustrated in Figure 4.2, where in three groups of AGA infants and in three groups of SGA infants TEWL during the first 4 weeks postnatally is compared with that on the first day after birth (regression curves). The clear change in TEWL indicates that the barrier function of the epidermis quickly improves[28].

There is also a linear relationship between the evaporation rate from the skin surface and the ambient relative humidity, with much higher evaporation rates at a low ambient humidity than at a high humidity (Figure 4.3).

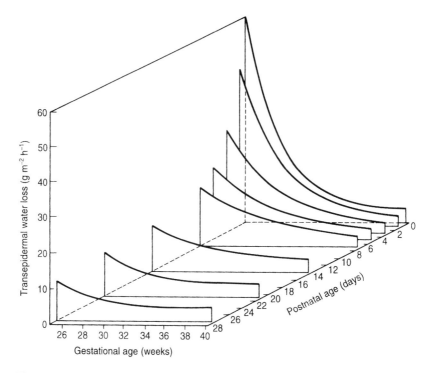

Figure 4.1 Transepidermal water loss in relation to gestational age at birth and at different postnatal ages in appropriate for gestational age infants. (From Hammarlund et al[28] with permission.)

The insensible water loss from the skin (IWL$_s$), as calculated from TEWL, body surface area and weight, is presented in Table 4.1. In infants born at 25–27 weeks of gestation IWL$_s$ decreases during the first week after birth, from 129 g kg^{-1} 24 h^{-1} to 43 g kg^{-1} 24 h^{-1} in an

Table 4.1 Mean insensible water loss through the skin (g kg^{-1} 24 h^{-1}) in appropriate for gestational age infants at an ambient relative humidity of 50%

Gestational age (weeks)	Mean birthweight (kg)	Postnatal age (days)			
		<1	3	7	28
25–27	0.860	129	71	43	24
28–30	1.340	42	32	24	15
31–36	2.110	12	12	12	7
37–41	3.600	7	6	6	7

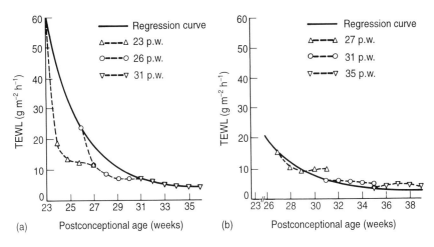

Figure 4.2 Transepidermal water loss (TEWL) in three groups of (a) appropriate for gestational age infants, and (b) small for gestational age infants during the first 4 weeks postnatally (dashed lines) compared with TEWL on the first day after birth (regression curves). Post-conceptional age (p.w.) was calculated as gestational age at birth minus 2 weeks plus postnatal age. (From Hammarlund et al[28] with permission.)

environment with an ambient humidity of 50%. At that ambient humidity, the water losses through the skin of these infants even exceed the fluid volume excreted as urine during the first day after birth.

IWL$_s$ and ambient humidity

Much less water is lost from the skin at an ambient humidity of 80% than at a low humidity (20%). At an ambient humidity of 20% a very preterm infant with a weight of 1 kg loses one-fifth of body weight during the first 24 hours after birth (205 g kg^{-1} 24 h^{-1}). In a very humid environment (80%) the same infant will lose only one-twentieth of body weight (53 g kg^{-1} 24 h^{-1}). The difference between these two extremes is 152 g kg^{-1} 24 h^{-1} [28,29]. Without good knowledge of the environmental conditions, it is very difficult to estimate insensible water loss early after birth in very preterm infants. There is a considerable difference between the amount of water that has to be given to replace the IWL$_s$ when the infant is nursed in an environment with an ambient relative humidity of 20% and that when it is nursed in a humidity of 80%. This is illustrated in Figure 4.4.

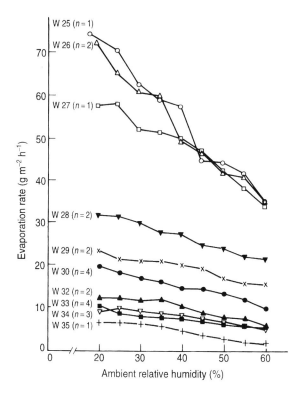

Figure 4.3 The relation between evaporation rate and ambient relative humidity in preterm appropriate for gestational age newborn infants in different gestational age groups. W, completed weeks of gestation. (From Hammarlund et al[26] with permission.)

Activity, temperature, phototherapy and care under radiant heaters

It is known that in fullterm infants TEWL increases considerably with activity, without the occurrence of visible sweating or an increase in body temperature[13], but there is limited knowledge about how activity and temperature influence the water loss from the skin surface in very preterm infants. In recently published studies in moderately preterm infants, no increase in IWL_s was found during phototherapy[30]. When preterm infants are nursed under a radiant heater the water loss from the skin can be higher if the relative humidity in the environmental air is low but there will be no increase due to the radiant energy itself[31].

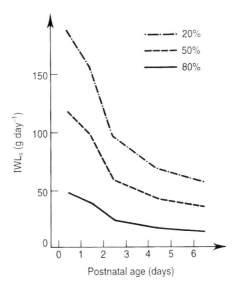

Figure 4.4 Insensible water loss from the skin (IWL$_s$) in relation to postnatal age in infants born at a gestational age of 25–27 weeks. Data are given for three different ambient humidities.

Water Loss from the Respiratory Tract

The respiratory water loss depends on the temperature and humidity of the inspired air and on the respiratory rate, the tidal volume, the dead space ventilation and the ability of the nose to dehumidify and cool the expiratory air[32,33]. In newborn fullterm infants at rest the respiratory water loss is 4.9 mg kg^{-1} min^{-1}, i.e. about 50% of the total insensible water loss, at an ambient air temperature of 32.5°C and an ambient humidity of 50%[32]. Respiratory water loss is also dependent on the ambient humidity[32]. Fullterm infants can increase their respiratory water loss markedly during activity[33] and when nursed in a warm environment[34]. An increase in the rate of breathing is accompanied by an increase in respiratory water loss. The same factors will probably influence the respiratory water loss in very preterm infants[35]. In very preterm infants inspiring a humidified gas in an incubator or through respirator tubing, the respiratory water loss is very low. The respiratory water loss will be zero if the gas the infant inspires is saturated with water at body temperature.

SUPPLY OF FLUIDS AND ELECTROLYTES

When infants are given nutrition and/or water early after birth the amount of fluid to be supplied has to be decided arbitrarily. Very wide variations in the recommended amounts to be given are encountered.

In fullterm infants, who normally have low insensible losses of water, corrections of the water balance can be made by increasing or decreasing the daily prescribed fluid supply. In preterm infants, who have high insensible water losses, dramatic losses of water, sometimes leading to severe hyperosmolality, have to be avoided. In a humid environment the insensible water loss is low and the supply of fluid can be kept low, i.e. 65–90 ml kg^{-1} day^{-1} during the first 3 days after birth. The body weight can then be allowed to decrease slowly while the necessary adjustments in interstitial water take place[13,29].

In preterm infants nursed in a dry environment, high insensible water losses have to be compensated for by supplying a larger volume of fluid. Larger administered fluid volumes, on the other hand, can lead to complications such as patent ductus arteriosus and necrotizing enterocolitis, and pulmonary and general oedema[36,37].

Electrolytes
It has previously been found that sodium excretion in the urine is higher in very preterm infants than in more mature infants and that this may lead to hyponatraemia[16] (for review see references 7 and 8). This has led to a recommendation that more sodium (3–4 mmol kg^{-1} day^{-1}) should be supplied in very preterm infants[38]. An increased solute load, however, may result in increased urine volumes and dehydration[9,16]. Bueva and Guignard[39] have suggested that even very preterm infants are able to maintain their sodium balance with a sodium intake of 1–2 mmol kg^{-1} day^{-1}.

Practical Aspects of Neonatal Water Balance

The following guidelines for fluid supply in preterm infants are recommended.

1. *Fluid supply during the first days after birth*
    Day 1: 65 ml kg^{-1}
    Day 2: 75 ml kg^{-1}
    Day 3: 90 ml kg^{-1}
    Days 4–7: Increase gradually up to 150 ml kg^{-1}
    All fluids given and removed should be noted.

2. *Additional rules for very preterm infants*
   (a) Body weight should be recorded accurately once or twice daily.
   (b) High ambient humidity (80–95%).
   (c) Every urine portion is to be tested for glucose, albumin and osmolality or specific gravity.
   (d) Daily analyses of serum osmolality, serum albumin and blood glucose, at least during the first 5 postnatal days.
   (e) Daily analyses of serum concentrations of sodium and potassium.

The basic prescription of fluid volumes may be changed if the plasma osmolality increases to above 300 mmol^{-1} l^{-1} and if the weight reduction exceeds 10–15%[29].

The type of fluid most frequently given to infants of all gestational ages during the first days after birth is glucose 100 mg ml^{-1} (10%) without any added electrolytes. In very preterm infants the glucose infusion may result in glucosuria and osmotic diuresis. If this occurs, the blood glucose level should be determined, and if it is high (>10 mmol l^{-1}), fluid with a lower glucose concentration should be given to achieve a normal blood glucose. Serum concentrations of sodium and potassium should be determined daily. Supplementation of electrolytes is usually not necessary during the first 2 days after birth. Subsequently, sodium 2–3 mmol kg^{-1} day^{-1} and potassium 1–2 mmol kg^{-1} day^{-1} may be needed to meet basal requirements.

Infants with gastrointestinal disorders or in need of surgery are only given total parenteral nutrition with glucose, lipids and amino acids. In most infants, oral or gavage feeding with maternal or banked breast milk can be started as soon as the infant is in a stable condition.

Even in extremely preterm infants gavage feeding with breast milk 0.5–1.5 ml kg^{-1} every second hour can be started a few hours after birth. If there is no or little gastric retention of fluid, the volume of breast milk given every second hour can be increased to 1–2 ml kg^{-1} on the second day and 2–4 ml kg^{-1} on the third day postnatally. The volume given by oral/gavage feeding is gradually increased until sufficient nutrients and energy are supplied. Usually 50% of the total fluid supply can be given orally or by gavage feeding on the 5th or 6th day after birth. In infants with a high or increasing serum osmolality or serum sodium concentration, 0.5–2 ml sterile water can be added to the volume given by gavage feeding until serum osmolality is normalized. This volume of water is added to the recommended daily fluid supply. In addition to the oral/gavage feeding and infusion of glucose, parenteral infusion of increasing volumes of a lipid emulsion and an amino acid solution are started within the first 3 days after birth, with careful monitoring of the blood glucose level, turbidity and the acid–base status. After extubation, oral/gavage feeding is withheld for 24 hours and the entire supply of fluid and nutrients is given parenterally.

Practical Applications of these Recommendations in Extremely Preterm Infants

To exemplify how the practical rules mentioned above can be applied in two groups of extremely preterm infants, we extracted data concerning fluid supply, weight and serum analyses of sodium and osmolality from the patient records for all infants born after 24 or 27 completed weeks of gestation. All consecutively born infants at 24 or 27 weeks of gestation at the Obstetric Unit of Uppsala University Hospital during 1992 and 1993 were included. Fifteen infants were born at a gestational age of 24 weeks and 11 of these survived. During the same period 17 infants were born at 27 weeks of gestation and 15 of these survived. They were all nursed in double walled incubators (Dräger 8000) at an ambient humidity of 80–85%. Information concerning the fluid supply to the surviving infants born after 24 weeks of gestation is presented in Figure 4.5. Here it is seen that the infants born at 24 weeks of gestation had a mean birthweight of 694 g (range 588–785 g). The postnatal weight loss was very small during the first 2 days after birth (5.9%). The lowest mean weight (605 g) was reached 6 days after birth. The maximal mean weight reduction was 12.8%. During the second week after birth there was a steady increase in weight to a mean weight of 655 g 14 days after birth. During the first 7 days after birth the total fluid supply was increased to about 150 ml kg^{-1} body weight (Figure 4.5a). Five days after birth one-third of the total fluid supply was given as enteral fluid, i.e. breast milk supplied by gavage feeding. From the 10th day after birth about half of the total fluid supply was given as breast milk in infants born at 24 weeks of gestation (Figure 4.5).

In infants born at a gestational age of 24 weeks, the mean serum osmolality (Figure 4.6) was very close to 300 mosm kg^{-1} over the first few days. Three out of 11 infants transiently had a serum osmolality exceeding 320 mosm kg^{-1}. The mean serum sodium concentration was close to 150 mmol l^{-1} during the first 2 days after birth. Later it was about 140 mmol l^{-1} (range 134–145 mmol l^{-1}).

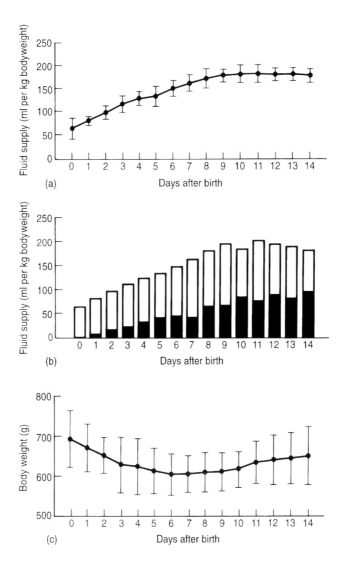

Figure 4.5 (a) Mean total fluid supply (±SD), with indication of (b) parenteral (□) and enteral (■) route of supply and (c) body weight, in relation to postnatal age, in infants born at a gestation of 24 weeks.

Because of hyperosmolality ($>300\ \mathrm{mosm}\ \mathrm{kg}^{-1}$), extra water was supplied with the breast milk (gavage feeding) during the first day after birth in one infant born at 24 weeks of gestation. During the second day after birth two infants received some extra sterilized water

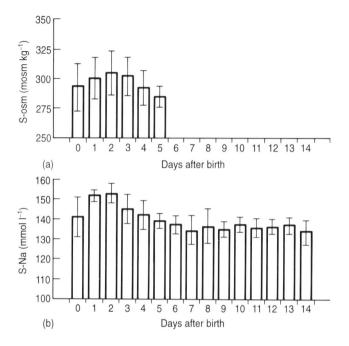

(a)

(b)

Figure 4.6 (a) Mean serum osmolality (S-osm ±SD) and (b) mean serum sodium concentration (S-Na ±SD) in 11 infants born at a gestational age of 24 weeks, in relation to postnatal age.

(2.5–6 ml). Three days after birth three infants received some extra sterilized water. No extra sodium was supplied during the first 2 days after birth. One infant was given an extra 2 mmol sodium during the third day after birth.

For comparison, data on weight and fluid supply are presented for infants born at 27 weeks of gestation (Figure 4.7). The mean body weight of 1000 g (range 695–1259 g) decreased to a lowest mean weight of 880 g on the 5th day after birth, i.e. a mean weight reduction of 12.0%. The mean body weight then increased and was 980 g 14 days after birth. The fluid supply in these infants (Figure 4.7a) was increased to about 150 ml kg^{-1} body weight on the 7th day after birth. Gavage feeding with breast milk was started immediately after birth and the volume of breast milk given by gavage feeding was more than 50% of the total fluid supply on the 7th day after birth (Figure 4.7a).

In infants born at 27 weeks of gestation the serum osmolality was a little lower than 300 mosm kg^{-1} during the first 5 days after birth, and

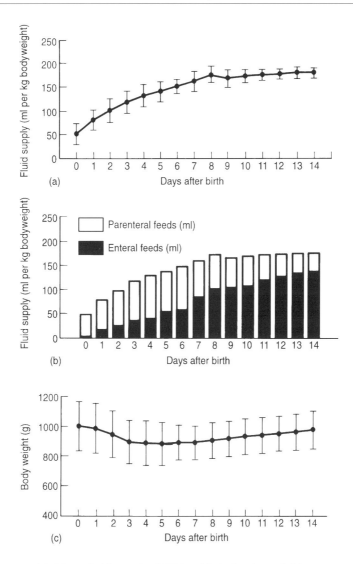

Figure 4.7 (a) Mean fluid supply (±SD), with indication of (b) parenteral (□) and enteral (■) route of supply and (c) body weight, in relation to postnatal age, in 15 infants born at a gestation of 27 weeks.

serum sodium was around 140 mmol l⁻¹. No infant had a serum osmolality exceeding 310 mosm kg⁻¹. No extra sodium was supplied during the first 3 days after birth. None of the infants born at 27 weeks of gestation were given any extra water supply.

CONCLUSION

Water balance in the most preterm newborn infants is best maintained, if excessive losses are to be prevented, by nursing the infants in a humid environment and by keeping them in good heat balance. Replacement fluids often contain solute, while the fluid lost is almost solute free, so rehydration may lead to hyperosmolality, with high sodium levels and often hyperglycaemia. From this presentation of data in infants born at 24 and 27 weeks of gestation it is clear that an acceptable water and electrolyte balance can be maintained by supplying moderate amounts of fluid and electrolytes while excessive losses of water through the transepidermal and respiratory routes are prevented by having a high environmental humidity in the incubator, and warm and humidified gas for ventilation of infants who need assisted ventilation. Enteral feeding is very well tolerated by these preterm infants and makes its easier to supply sufficient energy and nutrients.

Acknowledgements

Many of the results presented were obtained in studies supported by the Swedish Medical Research Council, grant 19X–4998.

REFERENCES

1. Smith FG, Nakmura KT, Segar JL and Robillard JE. Renal function in utero. In: Polin RA and Fox WF (eds) *Fetal and Neonatal Physiology*. London: Saunders, 1992:1187–1195.
2. Bland RD and Chapman DL. Absorption of liquid from the lungs at birth. In: Effros RM and Chang HK (eds) *Fluid and Solute Transport in the Airspaces of the Lungs*. New York: Marcel Dekker, 1994:303–322.
3. Olver RE. Fluid secretion and absorption in the fetus. In: Effros RM and Chang HK (eds) *Fluid and Solute Transport in the Airspaces of the Lungs*. New York: Marcel Dekker, 1994:281–302.
4. Barnes RJ. Water and mineral exchange between maternal and fetal fluids. In: Beard RW and Nathanielsz PW (eds) *Fetal Physiology and Medicine*. London: Saunders, 1976.
5. Friis-Hansen B. Changes in body water compartments during growth. *Acta Paediatr Scand Suppl* 1956;**110**.
6. Costarino AT and Baumgart S. Water as nutrition. In: Tsang RC, Lucas A, Uauy R and Zlotkin S (eds) *Nutritional Needs of the Preterm Infant*. Baltimore: Williams & Wilkins, 1992: 1–14.

7. Haycock GB and Aperia A. Salt and the newborn kidney. *Pediatr Nephrol* 1991;**5**:65–70.
8. Herin P and Aperia A. Neonatal kidney, fluids, and electrolytes. *Curr Opin Pediatr* 1994;**6**:154–157.
9. Herin P and Zetterström R. Sodium chloride and potassium needs in low-birth-weight infants. *Acta Paediatr Suppl* 1994;**405**:43–48.
10. Bauer K, Bovermann G, Roithmaier A, Götz M, Plölss A and Versmold HT. Body composition, nutrition, and fluid balance during the first two weeks of life in preterm neonates weighing less than 1500 grams. *J Pediatr* 1991;**118**:615–620.
11. Hey EN and Katz G. Evaporative water loss in the newborn baby. *J Physiol* 1969;**200**:605–619.
12. Harpin VA and Rutter N. Development of emotional sweating in the newborn infant. *Arch Dis Child* 1982;**57**:691–695.
13. Sedin G, Hammarlund K, Nilsson GE, Strömberg B and Öberg PÅ. Measurements of transepidermal water loss in newborn infants. *Clin Perinatol* 1985;**12**:79–99.
14. Coulthard MG and Hey EN. Effect of varying water intake on renal function in healthy preterm babies. *Arch Dis Child* 1985;**60**:614–620.
15. Costarino AT, Gruskay JA, Corcoran L, Polin RA and Baumgart S. Sodium restriction versus daily maintenance replacement in very low birth weight premature neonates: a randomized, blind therapeutic trial. *J Pediatr* 1992;**120**:99–106.
16. Vanpée M, Herin P, Zetterström R et al. Postnatal development of renal function in very low birthweight infants. *Acta Paediatr Scand* 1988; **77**:191–197.
17. Wilkins BH. Renal function in sick very low birthweight infants: 3. Sodium, potassium and water excretion. *Arch Dis Child* 1992;**67**:1154–1161.
18. Ekblad H, Kero P, Vuolteenaho O, Arjamaa O, Korvenranta H and Schaffer SG. Atrial natriuretic peptide in the preterm infant. Lack of correlation with natriuresis and diuresis. *Acta Pediatr* 1992;**81**:978–982.
19. Midgley J, Modi N, Littleton P, Carter N, Royston P and Smith A. Atrial natriuretic peptide, cyclic guanosine monophosphate and sodium excretion during postnatal adaptation in male infants below 34 weeks gestation with severe respiratory distress syndrome. *Early Hum Dev* 1992;**28**:145–154.
20. Pesonen E, Heldt GP, Merritt TA et al. Atrial natriuretic factor and pulmonary status in premature infants with respiratory distress syndrome; preliminary investigation. *Pediatr Pulmonol* 1993;**15**:362–364
21. Lemoh JN and Brooke OG. Frequency and weight of normal stools in infancy. *Arch Dis Child* 1979;**54**:719–720.
22. Patrick CH and Pittard WB. Stool water loss in very-low-birth-weight neonates. *Clin Pediatr* 1987;**27**:144–146.
23. Sedin G, Hammarlund K and Strömberg B. Transepidermal water loss in fullterm and preterm infants. *Acta Paediatr Scand Suppl* 1983;**305**:27–31.
24. Cartlidge Patrick HT and Rutter N. Skin barrier function. In: Polin RA and Fox WW (eds) *Fetal and Neonatal Physiology*. London: Saunders, 1992: 569–585.

25. Hammarlund K, Nilsson G, Öberg PÅ and Sedin G. Transepidermal water loss in newborn infants. I. Relation to ambient humidity and site of measurement and estimation of total transepidermal water loss. *Acta Paediatr Scand* 1977;**66:**553–562.

26. Hammarlund K and Sedin G. Transepidermal water loss in newborn infants. III. Relation to gestational age. *Acta Paediatr Scand* 1979; **68:**795–801.

27. Nilsson GE. Measurement of water exchange through the skin. *Med Biol Eng Comput* 1977;**15:**209–218.

28. Hammarlund K, Sedin G and Strömberg B. Transepidermal water loss in newborn infants. VIII. Relation to gestational age and post-natal age in appropriate and small for gestational age infants. *Acta Paediatr Scand,* 1983;**72:**721–728.

29. Sedin G, Hammarlund K, Riesenfeld T and Strömberg B. Optimal environment in very low birth weight infants <1500 g). Effect of humidity. In: Duc G (ed) *Controversial Issues in Neonatal Interventions.* New York: Thieme, 1989:109–122.

30. Kjartansson S, Hammarlund K and Sedin G. Insensible water loss from the skin during phototherapy in term and preterm infants. *Acta Paediatr* 1992;**81:**764–768.

31. Kjartansson S, Arsan S, Sjörs G, Hammarlund K and Sedin G. Water loss from the skin of term and preterm infants nursed under a radiant heater. *Pediatr Res,* 1995;**37:**233–238.

32. Riesenfeld T, Hammarlund K and Sedin G. Respiratory water loss in full-term infants on their first day after birth. *Acta Paediatr Scand* 1987; **76:**647–653.

33. Riesenfeld T, Hammarlund K and Sedin G. Respiratory water loss in relation to activity in fulltern infants on their first day after birth. *Acta Paediatr Scand* 1987;**76:**889–893.

34. Riesenfeld T, Hammarlund K and Sedin G. The effect of a warm environment on respiratory water loss in fulltern newborn infants on their first day after birth. *Acta Paediatr Scand* 1990;**79:**893–898.

35. Riesenfeld T, Hammarlund K and Sedin G. Respiratory water loss in relation to gestational age in infants on their first day after birth. *Acta Paediatr* 1995;**84:**1056–1059.

36. Bell EF, Warburton D, Stonestreet BS and Oh W. Effect of fluid administration on the development of symptomatic patent arteriosus and congestive heart failure in premature infants. *N Engl J Med* 1980;**302:**598–604.

37. Bell EF, Warburton D, Stonestree BS and Oh W. High-volume fluid intake predisposes premature infants to necrotising enterocolitis. *Lancet* 1979;**ii:**90.

38. Rees L, Shaw JCL, Brook CGD and Forsling ML. Hyponatraemia in the first week of life in preterm infants. Part II Sodium and water balance. *Arch Dis Child* 1984;**59:**423–429.

39. Bueva A and Guignard J-P. Renal function in preterm neonates. *Pediatr Res* 1994;**36:**572–577.

5

Outcome of Infants Born at Less than 26 Weeks Gestation

Victor Y.H. Yu, Elizabeth A. Carse and Margaret P. Charlton

INTRODUCTION

The limits of fetal and neonatal viability have changed dramatically since the mid-1970s. Previously, extremely low birthweight (ELBW, <1000 g) survivors were generally born relatively mature but growth retarded. With improved obstetric and neonatal care and a proactive attitude towards resuscitation at delivery and neonatal intensive care, an increasing number of liveborn infants delivered at 23–25 weeks gestation are surviving, as well as the occasional infant of 22 weeks. However, controversy and uncertainty remain regarding the obstetric management of the woman with threatened birth of an infant of extremely low gestation, and the neonatal management of such infants should they be born alive. Some obstetricians and neonatologists feel that, for these infants, the prospects of survival are so low and the proportion of survivors with severe disability is so high that life sustaining treatment should be withheld. The enormous expenditure from prolonged, high technology intensive care for such extremely preterm infants has also led to the debate on distributive justice in an economic climate where resources are scarce. Furthermore, concerns have been expressed that their improving survival may contribute substantially to an increasing number of severely disabled children within the community. The purpose of this chapter is to provide a contemporary knowledge base to assist readers in the decision making process for the infant of <26 weeks. This chapter will discuss the importance of determining gestational age; the prognosis for survival and subsequent neurodevelopmental outcome and health status; the risk factors for mortality and disability, and strategies which promise to enhance survival and quality of life; and the ethics of selective non-treatment as applied to extremely preterm infants.

DETERMINATION OF GESTATIONAL AGE AND FETAL WEIGHT

Birthweight-specific outcome data are useful for the neonatologist who can accurately measure the birthweight of an extremely preterm infant. However, estimates of fetal weight using ultrasonography vary within 10–15% of actual weight, depending on the biometric indices used to calculate fetal weight, amount of amniotic fluid, fetal presentation and lie, and the expertise of the operator[1]. It has been reported that obstetricians tended to underestimate birthweight, and the perinatal mortality of those with underestimated birthweight was significantly higher than those with correctly estimated birthweight[2]. Therefore, studies using gestational age as an independent variable influencing outcome are required to assist obstetricians, neonatologists and parents with their clinical decision making process when presented with the threatened birth of an extremely preterm infant. Menstrual history, corroborated by results of a first trimester pelvic examination, measurement of symphysis–fundus height and an early ultrasonographic examination, provides the best antenatal assessment of gestational age. More widespread use of early ultrasonography in pregnancy in recent years has made assessment of gestational age more reliable, and should encourage more cohort studies based on gestation rather than on birthweight. Postnatal assessment of gestational age is known to be unreliable in extremely preterm infants[3,4].

This chapter reviews data primarily derived from gestation cohorts, but where information is lacking, outcome of infants of <750–800 g is described. Although such infants are not exactly comparable with those of <26 weeks, the approximate mean birthweights for extremely preterm infants have been reported to be 500 g for 22 weeks, 600 g for 23 weeks, 700 g for 24 weeks, and 800 g for 25 weeks[5].

OUTCOME ACCORDING TO HOSPITAL BASED STUDIES

Survival

Reviews on the outcome of ELBW infants have confirmed that their survival rate has improved substantially since 1965 when such studies were first reported[6,7]. However, a survey of 23 hospitals in the United States published in 1986 reported that the survival rate in 716 infants of <26 weeks gestation was only about 10%, with virtually no improvement in survival between 1978 and 1983[8]. It therefore suggested that the better survival was achieved in the early 1980s only in the more mature infants who were >26 weeks among those who were ELBW. It was possible to obtain survival data of infants born at individual weeks of gestation below 26 weeks in 20 hospital based studies[9-26]. Gestational age is expressed in these studies in completed weeks; for example, the period 24 weeks and 0 days to 24 weeks and 6 days of gestation is referred to as '24 weeks'[5].

Table 5.1 shows an overall trend of improving survival for infants of <26 weeks from 1977 to 1993, especially in the more recent cohorts after introduction of surfactant replacement therapy[23-26]. However, close comparison between individual studies is not possible because of differences in the numerator and denominator used in these reports. A number of these studies include both inborn and outborn infants[17,19,22,23,26]. It is important to report outcome for infants born within the hospital (inborn) separately from those transported in after selective referral from other hospitals (outborn). Our own population based study of ELBW infants from the State of Victoria, Australia[27], and another from the McMaster Health Region in Ontario, Canada[28], have shown that only about half of these small infants born alive outside level III perinatal centres were referred for neonatal intensive care, and, with very few exceptions, those not transferred died. Although this practice of selective transfer had resulted in an apparently better survival rate in the subgroup of outborn infants referred for treatment, we have shown an association between suboptimal perinatal care prior to admission to the neonatal intensive care unit (NICU) of the perinatal centre and adverse neuro-developmental outcome[29]. Even for an inborn population, it is necessary to know whether only those infants born <26 weeks who remained alive long enough to be admitted to the NICU were included in the study, as this would mean exclusion of those livebirths who died in the delivery room because they failed to respond to resuscitation or resuscitation was withheld. The denominator used in

Table 5.1 Survival rate for infants of 22–25 weeks gestational age from hospital based studies

Authors	Year of birth	Survival data	Number of survivors			
			22 weeks	23 weeks	24 weeks	25 weeks
Herschel et al[9]	1977–1980	Neonatal	—	—	2/7 (29)	3/28 (11)
Dillon and Egan[10]	1977–1980	Hospital	—	—	4/11 (36)	6/16 (38)
Yu et al[11]	1977–1981	2 years	—	—	8/22 (36)	7/23 (30)
Kitchen et al[12]	1977–1982	Hospital	—	—	2/27 (7)	11/54 (20)
Milligan et al[13]	1979–1982	Hospital	—	1/7 (14)	9/23 (39)	28/44 (64)
Nwaesei et al[14]	1980–1982	Hospital	—	0/7 (0)	1/10 (10)	5/13 (38)
Yu et al[15]	1981–1984	2 years	—	2/19 (11)	7/23 (30)	6/25 (24)
Amon[16]	1981–1985	Hospital	—	5/73 (7)	7/63 (11)	31/66 (47)
Whyte et al[17]	1982–1987	Hospital	—	0/24 (0)	16/52 (31)	63/90 (70)
Hack and Fanaroff[18]	1982–1988	1 year	1/29 (3)	3/37 (8)	8/51 (16)	42/80 (53)
Cooke[19]	1980–1989	3 years	—	—	8/64 (13)	65/111 (59)
Doyle et al[20]	1984–1986	Hospital	—	—	0/17 (0)	8/26 (31)
Yu et al[21]	1977–1986	Hospital	—	2/30 (7)	14/47 (30)	19/61 (31)
Ishizuka[22]	1986–1988	1 year	5/7 (71)	49/60 (82)	—	—
Fujimura*	1986–1990	1 year	—	7/13 (54)	29/43 (67)	34/46 (74)
Silver et al[23]	1987–1989	Neonatal	—	—	17/47 (36)	—
Yu†	1987–1992	2 years	—	1/18 (6)	9/39 (23)	26/41 (63)
Allen et al[24]	1988–1991	6 months	—	6/36 (17)	19/34 (56)	31/39 (80)
Nishida and Ishizuka[25]	1990	Neonatal	3/36 (8)	43/118 (36)	—	—
Cooke[26]	1990–1993	Hospital	—	6/17 (35)	23/40 (58)	21/36 (58)

Values in parentheses are percentages.
* Personal communication.
† Unpublished data.

a number of the published studies was admissions to the NICU[19,22,25,26]. Several of the reports excluded infants with major or lethal malformations[9,14,17]. There was also variable reporting of survival duration, some studies reporting neonatal survival (28 days), some survival to discharge, and some late survival from 6 months to 3 years. Neonatal survival is not an adequate indicator of outcome in these small infants because a significant proportion of deaths is occurring after the first month of life, directly or indirectly related to their extremely preterm birth[30].

The overall 2 year survival for infants born alive at 23–26 weeks at Monash Medical Centre over the 16 year period 1977–1992 was 30%. No infant born at 22 weeks survived. We did not observe an obvious trend in improvement of survival in more recent years for

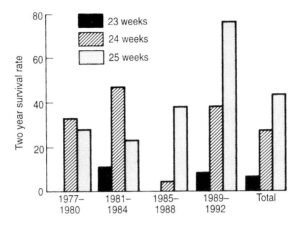

Figure 5.1 Two year survival rate of infants born at 23–25 weeks gestation in Monash Medical Centre over the 16 year period 1977–1992.

infants born at 23 and 24 weeks (Figure 5.1). However, the survival rate for infants born at 25 weeks has more than doubled over this study period (P=0.0003), and 22 (76%) of 29 such infants born in 1989–1992 survived to 2 years.

Disability

Improved survival in infants of <26 weeks, especially in those of 25 weeks, has led to renewed concern over the prevalence of their disability. Available data on neurodevelopmental outcome of these extremely preterm infants are sparse (Table 5.2). Complete follow up of survivors was achieved in all eight reports, except one which had an attrition rate of 5%[17]. Not all studies have the same definition of disability. Commonly used criteria included a mental developmental index (MDI) on the Bayley Scales of Infant Development <69, cerebral palsy, blindness and sensorineural deafness requiring aids[1-3]. A developmental quotient <85 was used in other studies[4,7] and hydrocephalus and uncontrolled epilepsy were also included in the definition of disability[4,5]. Except for a high disability rate in a handful of survivors of 22 weeks reported in one study[22], the overall prevalence of disability reported among 340 survivors of 23–25 weeks from these studies was 30%.

At Monash Medical Centre, 17 (24%) of 70 survivors of 23–25 weeks born in 1977–1992 had one or more disabilities diagnosed at 2

Table 5.2 Severe disability rate for infants of 22–25 weeks gestational age from hospital based studies

Authors	Year of birth	Age at assessment (years)	Number with disability			
			22 weeks	23 weeks	24 weeks	25 weeks
Yu et al[11]	1977–1981	2	—	—	1/8 (13)	4/7 (57)
Nwaesei et al[14]	1980–1982	2	—	—	0/1	2/5 (40)
Yu et al[15]	1981–1984	2	—	1/2 (50)	1/7 (14)	2/6 (33)
Whyte et al[17]	1982–1987	2	—	—	11/14 (79)	20/59 (34)
Cooke[19]	1980–1989	3	—	—	3/8 (38)	12/46 (26)
Ishizuka[22]	1986–1988	?	4/5 (80)	20/49 (41)	—	—
Fujimura*	1986–1990	?	—	3/6 (50)	13/27 (48)	10/32 (31)
Yu†	1985–1992	2	—	0/1	3/10 (30)	10/33 (30)

Values in parentheses are percentages.
* Personal communication.
† Unpublished data.

years. No clear trend emerged from available data that the prevalence of disability is inversely proportional to gestational age for infants of <26 weeks. With respect to specific impairments, 20% had developmental delay, 14% had cerebral palsy, 6% had sensorineural deafness requiring aids, and 1% had bilateral blindness. Our finding that cognitive impairment, rather than cerebral palsy, was more common in this extremely preterm group was similarly reported in a Canadian study[17]. Although in our experience the rate of blindness induced by retinopathy of prematurity (ROP) had remained unchanged over a 12 year period, we did observe an increase in overall prevalence of ROP[31]. We have reported that among infants of 23–25 weeks 71% had ROP, 33% had ROP of stage 3 or worse, and 13% had at least one blind eye[31].

Although a majority of extremely preterm survivors may be free from disability, they experience more subtle forms of morbidity, including behaviour problems, which can produce serious psychological and educational sequelae in the longer term. These disorders manifest at school age with learning difficulties and problems with attention, perception, sequencing, language and organization of motor performance. Data from Monash Medical Centre have shown that the attention deficit was associated with a significantly lower MDI on the Bayley score[32]; more muscle tone disorders, minor physical and neurological disabilities, and poorer visual tracking, visual motor coordination and gross and fine motor coordination at 2 years[33]; more aggressiveness and less ability to cope with frustration at 5 years[34]; and significantly worse verbal, performance and full scale intelligence quotient on the Weschler Preschool and Primary Scale of Intelligence (WPPSI) at 5 years[35]. In a study from the United States, children with birthweights <750 g were reported to have poorer academic achievement and social skills, and more behavioural and attention problems at school age[36].

Health Status and Growth

Continuing health problems in extremely preterm infants may interact with their neurodevelopmental disability to worsen outcome, through diminished participation in appropriate activities, recurrent hospitalization, and school absences later in childhood. We have reported that 58% of children with birthweights <800 g born in 1977–1983 required rehospitalization in the first 2 years. When compared with normal birthweight children in the State of Victoria, the relative risk for rehospitalization was 3.2[37]. Their three most common medical problems experienced in the first 2 years were otitis media (66% of children), wheezy bronchitis (43%) and gastroenteritis (31%). Aural ventilation tube insertion (grommets) was required in 22% and inguinal herniorrhaphy in 10% of these children. Their health status improved between 2 and 5 years, when their rehospitalization rate and total hospital days were reduced[38]. Their three most common medical problems experienced at 2–5 years were otitis media (45% of children), tonsillitis (39%) and asthma (26%). In the United States it has been shown that by 6 years of age, 82% of ELBW children were considered by their parents to have good or excellent health, compared with 81% of control children born at term[39].

Head circumference measurements in children with birthweights <800 g were comparable with those of normal birthweight children, but about half of the children remained below the 10th percentile in weight and height at 2 years[37]. There was some catch-up in physical growth between 2 and 5 years but 42% remained below the 3rd percentile for weight and 19% for height at 5 years[38]. Other studies have reported that ELBW infants remained disadvantaged with respect to physical growth at 6–8 years of age[36,40]. The combined impact of neurodevelopmental disability and continuing health problems has important implications for how parents view their child and react to apparent vulnerability[41].

OUTCOME ACCORDING TO POPULATION BASED STUDIES

Population based studies on the outcome of extremely preterm infants from a designated region, rather than from a single hospital, are essential if the overall efficacy of perinatal care services is to be determined. Selection bias precludes results of hospital based studies from being extrapolated to a geographical region, and population based studies are necessary for the proper evaluation of neonatal intensive care programmes. Intensive perinatal–neonatal care cannot be established in all hospitals with a maternity unit to serve every high risk infant born within a geographically defined region, and such resources are concentrated in select level III perinatal centres. In the State of Victoria, which has an area of 87 000 square miles (225 300 km²) and 66 000 annual births in about 180 hospitals with a maternity unit, we endeavour to identify most high risk pregnancies through a comprehensive antenatal care programme, following which the fetus is transferred in utero to one of three level III perinatal centres for continued management. For the remaining high risk infants born outside a perinatal centre, a regional Newborn Emergency Transport Service has been established in the State of Victoria to transfer critically ill infants to an NICU for treatment.

Population based data are available from the State of Victoria on cohorts of ELBW infants since 1979. In addition to our own regional cohort data, two British studies have reported the outcome for children born at 24 and 25 weeks from a geographically defined area[42–44]. Table 5.3 shows that, although the survival rates were comparable between studies, the severe disability rate in our study was lower than that in the British studies. Our previous regional cohort studies have

Table 5.3 Outcome data for infants born at 24 and 25 weeks from population based studies

Authors	Year of birth	Age seen (years)	24 weeks		25 weeks	
			Survival	Disability	Survival	Disability
Wariyar et al[42]	1983	2	1/19 (5)	0/1	6/22 (27)	2/6 (33)
Johnson et al[43]	1984–1986	4	5/60 (8)	3/5 (60)	9/45 (20)	4/9 (44)
VICS[44]	1985–1987	5	10/86 (12)	1/10 (10)	31/109 (28)	4/31 (13)

Values in parentheses are percentages.
Definition of disability: ref. 42 – Griffiths' <70, severe cerebral palsy, deafness, vision <6/30;
ref. 43 – Griffiths' <70, severe cerebral palsy, deafness, blindness;
ref. 44 – WPPSI-R <70, severe cerebral palsy, blindness.

demonstrated that not only did inborn ELBW infants have a significantly higher survival rate compared with those who were outborn, they also had a significantly lower severe disability rate, three times less than that in outborn infants at 8 years of age[45]. We have also reported an improvement in both survival and disability rates in a regional cohort of ELBW infants, associated with a significant increase in the proportion of ELBW infants born within our perinatal centres[46]. Over the period 1985–1987 almost 90% of our extremely preterm cohort were born within one of the three perinatal centres in the State of Victoria[44]. A substantially lower proportion of inborn infants in the British studies[42,43] may account for the comparatively better neurodevelopmental outcome in the Australian study. Concerns that increasing survival rates for extremely preterm children would lead to an increase in the proportion or absolute number of severely disabled children in the community are not supported by our population based study in the State of Victoria[46].

STRATEGIES TO IMPROVE OUTCOME

Perinatal Factors Influencing Outcome

Future improvement in outcome of extremely preterm infants depends on the identification of risk factors that adversely affect survival and disability, as this would enable the development of effective strategies to obviate such unfavourable influences. Four studies are available in the literature, which reported an analysis of perinatal factors in a large inborn cohort of ELBW or extremely preterm infants to determine those factors which were significantly associated with death or disability[12,47-49]. Perinatal factors found to be significantly associated with death included antepartum haemorrhage, multiple pregnancy, breech presentation, absence of labour before delivery, absence of antenatal corticosteroid therapy, low Apgar score, male sex, hypothermia, systemic hypotension, severe respiratory distress syndrome (RDS), persistent pulmonary hypertension, sepsis, grade III or IV intraventricular haemorrhage and absence of postnatal surfactant therapy. Perinatal factors found to be significantly associated with disability among survivors included antepartum haemorrhage, absence of antenatal corticosteroid therapy, male sex, severe RDS, sepsis, grade III and IV intraventricular haemorrhage and hydrocephalus requiring ventriculoperitoneal shunting.

Our experience at Monash Medical Centre also suggested a number of additional factors increased the risk of death and/or disability in such high risk infants: transfer in utero after onset of preterm labour as compared with before onset of preterm labour[50], severe pre-eclampsia[51], pulmonary air leak[52], protracted seizures[53], periventricular haemorrhage and leucomalacia[54,55], and postnatal growth failure[56]. However, relative contributions to mortality or developmental disability of specific perinatal risk factors do vary between hospitals[57,58] where different strategies would be required to improve outcome.

The effect of the mode of delivery on outcome remains controversial. Little evidence was found from mortality or morbidity data to support routine delivery of infants of borderline viability by caesarean section[12,59,60]. It has been recommended that, for all infants <24 weeks and most infants of 24 weeks, caesarean section should not be performed for fetal distress and is indicated only for the mother's health[61]. However, caesarean section is considered an acceptable mode of delivery if the 25 weeks fetus is compromised during labour[61].

Antenatal Corticosteroid Therapy

Although antenatal corticosteroid therapy has been proven to be effective in improving neonatal mortality and morbidity after preterm delivery[62], only 10–20% of extreme preterm deliveries have been reported to occur after a full course of steroid therapy[63,64]. Evidence is available to suggest that it remains effective in reducing the incidence of RDS at 26–31 weeks[62,64], but insufficient numbers <26 weeks had received antenatal corticosteroids in published studies to be certain. Even if the prevalence of RDS is not decreased significantly, antenatal corticosteroids have been shown to be beneficial in reducing the severity of lung disease and prevalence of severe intraventricular haemorrhage in extremely preterm infants[65]. It has been reported that the addition of thyrotrophin releasing hormone to antenatal corticosteroid therapy reduced further the prevalence of RDS and mortality in preterm infants[66], but benefits among those <26 weeks have not been adequately studied.

Postnatal Surfactant Therapy

Surfactant replacement therapy has significantly reduced mortality from RDS in preterm infants[67] but little information is available on its effect in extremely preterm infants. One randomized clinical trial using synthetic surfactant failed to demonstrate increased survival in infants of 500–600 g[68], while another using bovine surfactant demonstrated an increased survival rate and a decreased disability rate in infants of 600–750 g[69]. Two non-randomized studies also reported that the use of surfactant was associated with improved survival in infants of 23–25 weeks and 500–749 g respectively[70,71]. Nevertheless, follow up studies on such extremely preterm survivors from the post-surfactant era are required, as concerns remain on the quality of life among those currently born at 23–24 weeks[24]. The suggested additive effect when antenatal corticosteroids and postnatal surfactant are used together[72] requires confirmation in extremely preterm infants.

Socioenvironmental Factors

Although considerable research has gone into the identification of medical risk factors affecting outcome and into efforts to improve the quality of perinatal–neonatal care, it is becoming increasing evident that socioenvironmental risk factors are as important, if not more so, in influencing early childhood development and cognitive functioning in preterm infants. Low levels of parenting capability[73], parental education[74], occupation[33,35] and socioeconomic status[75] are associated with significantly worse mental performance and cognitive function among preterm survivors, especially evident after 3 years of age[74]. A randomized clinical trial of home visits, parent support groups and a systematic educational programme provided in specialized child development centres has shown that such early intervention enhances the cognitive, behavioural and health status of preterm infants[76]. Data are not available on whether community efforts to improve the social, educational and economic environment of the families of infants born at <26 weeks are effective in improving their quality of life.

ETHICS OF SELECTIVE NON-TREATMENT

Among both obstetricians[77] and neonatologists[78] there is a tendency to underestimate the potential for survival and overestimate the risks of disability for extremely preterm infants. As a result, many of these livebirths were left to die through withholding of resuscitation or neonatal intensive care. If clinicians believe that the infant has little prospect for survival, their management would be less than optimal and they may in fact be creating a self-fulfilling prophecy. Failure to treat could violate the principle of patient centred beneficence, which requires the clinician to make every possible effort to benefit the infant. However, because so few infants born at <23 weeks are expected to live, it has been recommended that most should be offered palliative care only, and active treatment should be initiated only at the request of fully informed parents or if it appears that the gestational age has been underestimated[61]. As it is difficult to be certain of the prognosis at the time of birth for infants of 24 weeks, most of them should be offered resuscitation, and neonatal intensive care should be promptly initiated[79]. The attending clinician should discuss with the parents the need for flexibility in deciding to initiate or withhold treatment, depending on the infant's condition at birth. Resuscitation should be attempted for all infants of 25 weeks. Only in the event that the subsequent clinical course indicates that further curative efforts are futile or lack compensating benefit should life support measures be discontinued and palliative care, which provides symptomatic relief and comfort, be introduced. The attending neonatologist has the primary role as advocate for the infant and medical advisor to the parents, while the parents act as surrogates for their infant. The shift in emphasis from curative to palliative treatment requires medical consensus among all those involved in the care of the infant, and consent from the parents who are closely involved in this widely shared decision making process. The policy of selective treatment or non-treatment has been termed an 'individualized prognostic strategy'[80], and has received endorsement from the United States[81], Canada[61], United Kingdom[82] and Australia[83].

Failure to implement selective non-treatment for infants of <26 weeks in whom a situation of inherent uncertainty exists regarding outcome could violate the moral principle of non-maleficence (which mandates foremost that the clinician do no harm) and also of distributive justice (which compels appropriate allocation of finite resources). We reported that the costs per survivor born in 1985–1987 at 600–699 g and 700–799 g were $A131 690 and $A113 080 respectively[84]. Their costs per additional quality adjusted life year gained were $A6450 and $A5760 respectively. These cost : utility ratios are one-tenth of those published for an early-1970 cohort from Canada[85], which in themselves already demonstrated better value for money compared with coronary bypass surgery, peritoneal dialysis and haemodialysis[86]. Currently, neonatal intensive care for extremely preterm infants is estimated to be more cost effective than bone marrow transplant (2×), kidney transplant (3×), heart transplant (5×), liver transplant (8×), renal dialysis (9×), coronary bypass surgery (26×) and coronary care (40×). This requires confirmation using a recently proposed measure of 'health related quality of life', which allows direct and accurate comparison of neonatal intensive care with other health care programmes[87]. A strategy for selective treatment or non-treatment will assist containment of costs. Although it may result in a modest rise in mortality, significant reduction in the number of survivors with severe disability would ensue. Some extremely preterm infants will die who might otherwise have survived, but many others will be saved from unnecessary suffering. For the infant born at <26 weeks, compassion and justice is the recommended alternative to technological imperative.

REFERENCES

1. Mills MD, Nageotte MP, Elliot JP et al. Reliability of ultrasonographic formulary in the prediction of fetal weight and survival of very-low-birthweight infants. *Am J Obstet Gynecol* 1990;**163:**1568–1574.
2. Paul RH, Koh KS and Monfared AH. Obstetric factors influencing outcome in infants weighing 1000 to 1500 grams. *Am J Obstet Gynecol* 1979;**133:**503–508.
3. Spinnato JA, Sibai BM, Shaver DC and Anderson GD. Inaccuracy of Dubowitz gestational age in low birth weight infants. *Obstet Gynecol* 1984;**63:**491–495.
4. Sanders M, Allen M, Alexander GR et al. Gestational age assessment in preterm neonates weighing less than 1500 grams. *Pediatrics* 1991;**88:**542–546.
5. *International Classification of Disease*, 10th revision. Geneva: World Health Organization 1992.
6. Yu VYH. Survival and neurodevelopmental outcome of preterm infants. In: Yu VYH and Wood EC (eds) *Prematurity*. Edinburgh: Churchill Livingstone, 1987:223–245.
7. Nishida H. Outcome of infants born preterm, with special emphasis on extremely low birthweight infants. In: Rice GE and Brennecke SP (eds) *Preterm Labor and Delivery*. London: Baillière Tindall, 1993:611–631.
8. Sell EJ. Outcome of very very low birth weight infants. *Clin Perinatol* 1986;**13:**451–460.
9. Herschel M, Kennedy JL Jr, Kayne HL, Henry M and Cetruilo CL. Survival of infants born at 24 to 28 weeks' gestation. *Obstet Gynecol* 1982;**60:**154–158.
10. Dillon WP and Egan EA. Aggressive obstetric management in late second trimester deliveries. *Obstet Gynecol* 1981;**58:**685–690.
11. Yu VYH, Orgill AA, Bajuk B and Astbury J. Survival and 2-year outcome of extremely preterm infants. *Br J Obstet Gynaecol* 1984;**91:**640–646.
12. Kitchen WH, Ford GW, Doyle LW et al. Cesarean section or vaginal delivery at 24 to 28 weeks' gestation: comparison of survival and neonatal and two-year morbidity. *Obstet Gynecol* 1985;**66:**149–157.

13. Milligan JE, Shennan AT and Hoskin EM. Perinatal intensive care: Where and how to draw the line. *Am J Obstet Gynecol* 1984;**148:**499–503.

14. Nwaesei CG, Young DC, Byrne JM et al. Preterm birth at 23 to 26 weeks' gestation: is active obstetric management justified? *Am J Obstet Gynecol* 1987;**157:**890–897.

15. Yu VYH, Loke HL, Bajuk B, Szymonowicz W, Orgill AA and Astbury J. Prognosis for infants born at 23 to 28 weeks' gestation. *BMJ* 1986; **293:**1200–1203.

16. Amon E. Limits of fetal viability. Obstetric considerations regarding the management and delivery of the extremely premature baby. *Obstet Gynecol Clin North Am* 1988;**15:**321–338.

17. Whyte HE, Fitzhardinge PM, Shennan AT, Lennox K, Smith L and Lacy J. Extreme immaturity: outcome of 568 pregnancies of 23–26 weeks' gestation. *Obstet Gynecol* 1993;**82:**1–7.

18. Hack M and Fanaroff AA. Outcomes of extremely low birth weight infants between 1982 and 1988. *N Engl J Med* 1989;**321:**1642–1647.

19. Cooke RWI. Factors affecting survival and outcome at 3 years in extremely preterm infants. *Arch Dis Child* 1994;**71:**F28–31.

20. Doyle LW, Murton LJ and Kitchen WH. Increasing the survival of extremely immature (24 to 28 weeks' gestation) infants – at what cost? *Med J Aust* 1989;**150:**558–568.

21. Yu VYH, Gomez JM, Shah V and McCloud PI. Survival prospects of extremely preterm infants: a 10-year experience in a single perinatal center. *Am J Perinatol* 1992;**9:**164–169.

22. Ishizuka Y. Long term survival of infants born less than 500 grams or less than 24 weeks gestation. *J Jpn Pediatr Soc* 1990;**94:**841–844.

23. Silver RK, MacGregor SN, Farrell EE, Ragin A, Davis C and Socol ML. Perinatal factors influencing survival at twenty-four weeks' gestation. *Am J Obstet Gynecol* 193;**168:**1724–1731.

24. Allen MC, Donohue PK and Dusman AE. The limit of viability – neonatal outcome of infants born at 22 to 25 weeks' gestation. *N Engl J Med* 1993;**329:**1597–1601.

25. Nishida H and Ishizuka Y. Survival rate of extremely low birthweight infants and its effect on the amendment of the eugenic protection act in Japan. *Acta Paediatr Jpn* 1992;**34:**612–616.

26. Cooke RWI. Antenatal management and outcome in micronates. *Ross Special Conference: Hot Topics '94 in Neonatology.* Abbott Laboratories: Columbus, OH, 1994:350–351.

27. Kitchen WH, Campbell N, Drew JH, Murton LJ, Roy RND and Yu VYH. Provision of perinatal services and survival of extremely low birthweight infants in Victoria. *Med J Aust* 1983;**2:**314–318.

28. Saigal S, Rosenbaum P, Stoskopf B and Sinclair JC. Outcome in infants 501 to 1000 g birthweight delivered to residents of the McMaster Health Region. *J Pediatr* 1984;**105:**969–976.

29. Kitchen W, Ford G, Orgill AA et al. Outcome of infants of birthweight 500–999 g: a regional study of 1979–1980 births. *J Paediatr* 1984;**104:**921–927.

30. Yu VYH, Watkins A and Bajuk B. Neonatal and postneonatal mortality in very low birthweight infants. *Arch Dis Child* 1984;**59:**987–989.

31. Yu VYH, Lim CT and Downe LM. A 12-year experience of retinopathy of prematurity in infants ≤28 weeks gestation or ≤1000 g birthweight. *J Paediatr* Child Health 1990;**26:**205–208.

32. Astbury J, Orgill AA, Bajuk B and Yu VYH. Determinants of developmental performance in very low birthweight survivors at 1 and 2 years of age. *Dev Med Child Neurol* 1983;**25:**709–716.

33. Astbury J, Orgill AA, Bajuk B and Yu VYH. Neonatal and neurodevelopmental significance of behaviour in very low birthweight children. *Early Hum Dev* 1985;**11:**113–121.

34. Astbury J, Bajuk B, Orgill AA, Szymonowicz W and Yu VYH. The relationship of 2 year behaviour to neurodevelopmental outcome at 5 years in very low birthweight survivors. *Dev Med Child Neurol* 1987;**29:**370–379.

35. Astbury J, Orgill AA, Bajuk B and Yu VYH. Neurodevelopmental outcome, growth and health of extremely low birthweight survivors: how soon can we tell? *Dev Med Child Neurol* 1990;**32:**582–589.

36. Hack M, Taylor HG, Klein N, Eiben R, Schatschneider C and Mecuri-Minich N. School-age outcomes in children with birth weights under 750 g. *N Engl J Med* 1994;**331:**753–759.

37. Bowman E and Yu VYH. Continuing morbidity in extremely low birthweight infants. *Early Hum Dev* 1989;**18:**165–174.

38. Yu VYH, Manlapaz ML, Tobin J, Carse EA, Charlton MP and Gore JR. Improving health status in extremely low birthweight children between two and five years. *Early Hum Dev* 1992;**30:**229–239.

39. Teplin SW, Burchinal M, Johnson-Martin N, Humphry RA and Kraybill EN. Neurodevelopmental, health, and growth status at age 6 years of children with birth weights less than 1001 grams. *J Pediatr* 1991; **118:**768–777.

40. Saigal S, Szatmari P, Rosenbaum P, Campbell D and King S. Cognitive abilities and school performance of extremely low birth weight children and matched term control children at age 8 years: a regional study. *J Pediatr* 1991;**118:**751–760.

41. Perrin EC, West PD and Culley BS. Is my child normal yet? Correlates of vulnerability. *Pediatrics* 1989;**83:**355–363.

42. Wariyar U, Richmond S and Hey E. Pregnancy outcome at 24–31 weeks' gestation: neonatal survivors. *Arch Dis Child* 1989;**64:**678–686.

43. Johnson A, Townshend P, Yudkin P, Bull D and Wilkinson AR. Functional abilities at age 4 years of children born before 29 weeks of gestation. *BMJ* 1993;**306:**1715–1718.

44. Victorian Infant Collaborative Study Group. Outcome to five years of age of children 24–26 weeks' gestational age born in the State of Victoria. *Med J Aust* 1995;**163:**11–14.

45. Victorian Infant Collaborative Study Group. Eight year outcome in infants with birthweight 500 to 999 gm: continued regional study of 1979 and 1980 births. *J Pediatr* 1991;**118:**761–767.

46. Victorian Infant Collaborative Study Group. Impact of improved care for infants of birthweight under 1000 g. *Arch Dis Child* 1991;**66**:765–769.

47. Shennan AT, Milligan JE and Hoskin EM. Perinatal factors associated with death or handicap in very preterm infants. *Am J Obstet Gynecol* 1985; **151**:231–238.

48. Yu VYH, Downe L, Astbury J, Orgill AA and Bajuk B. Perinatal factors associated with adverse outcome in extremely low birthweight infants. *Arch Dis Child* 1986;**61**:554–558.

49. Msall ME, Buck GM, Rogers BT et al. Multivariate risks among extremely premature infants. *J Perinatol* 1994;**14**:41–47.

50. Yu VYH, Wong PY, Bajuk B, Orgill AA and Astbury J. Outcome of extremely low birthweight infants. *Br J Obstet Gynaecol* 1986;**93**:162–170.

51. Szymonowicz W and Yu VYH. Severe pre-eclampsia and the very low birthweight infant. *Arch Dis Child* 1987;**62**:712–716.

52. Yu VYH, Wong PY, Bajuk B and Szymonowicz W. Pulmonary air leak in extremely low birthweight infants. *Arch Dis Child* 1986;**61**:239–241.

53. Watkins A, Szymonowicz W, Jin X and Yu VYH. Significance of seizures in the very low birthweight infant. *Dev Med Child Neurol* 1988;**30**:170–180.

54. Catto-Smith AG, Yu VYH, Bajuk B, Orgill AA and Astbury J. Effect of neonatal periventricular hemorrhage on neurodevelopmental outcome. *Arch Dis Child* 1985;**60**:8–11.

55. Szymonowicz W, Yu VYH, Bajuk B and Astbury J. Neurodevelopmental outcome of periventricular hemorrhage and leukomalacia in infants 1250 grams or less at birth. *Early Hum Dev* 1986;**14**:1–7.

56. Astbury J, Orgill AA, Bajuk B and Yu VYH. Sequelae of growth failure in appropriate for gestational age very low birthweight infants. *Dev Med Child Neurol* 1986;**28**:472–479.

57. Bajuk B, Kitchen WH, Lissenden JV and Yu VYH. Perinatal factors affecting survival of very low birthweight infants – a study from two hospitals. *Aust Paediatr J* 1981;**17**:277–280.

58. Kitchen WH, Yu VYU, Orgill AA et al. Collaborative study of very low birth weight infants. Correlation of handicap with risk factors. *Am J Dis Child* 1983;**137**:555–559.

59. Yu VYH, Bajuk B, Cutting D, Orgill AA and Astbury J. Effect of mode of delivery on outcome of very low birthweight infants. *Br J Obstet Gynaecol* 1984;**9**:633–639.

60. Yu VYH, Loke HL, Bajuk B, Szymonowicz W, Orgill AA and Astbury J. Outcome of singleton infants delivered vaginally or by caesarean section at 23 to 28 weeks' gestation. *Aust NZ J Obstet Gynaecol* 1987;**27**:196–200.

61. Fetus and Newborn Committee, Canadian Paediatric Society; Maternal–Fetal Medicine Committee, Society of Obstetricians and Gynaecologists of Canada. Management of the women with threatened birth of an infant of extremely low gestational age. *Can Med Assoc J* 1994;**151**:547–553.

62. Crowley P, Chalmers I and Keirse MJNC. The effects of corticosteroid administration before preterm delivery: an overview of the evidence from controlled trials. *Br J Obstet Gynaecol* 1990;**97**:11–25.

63. Yu VYH, Bajuk B, Orgill AA and Astbury J. Viability of infants born at 24 to 26 weeks gestation. *Ann Acad Med* 1985;**14:**563–571.

64. Maher JE, Cliver SP, Goldenberg RL et al. The effect of corticosteroid therapy in the very premature infant. *Am J Obstet Gynecol* 1994; **170:**869–873.

65. Garite TJ, Rumney PJ, Briggs GG et al. A randomized, placebo-controlled trial of betamethasone for the prevention of respiratory distress syndrome at 24 to 28 weeks' gestation. *Am J Obstet Gynecol* 1992;**166:**645–651.

66. Knight DB, Liggins GC and Wealthall SR. A randomized, controlled trial of antepartum thyrotropin-releasing hormone and betamethasone in the prevention of respiratory disease in preterm infants. *Am J Obstet Gynecol* 1994;**171:**11–16.

67. Jobe AH. Pulmonary surfactant therapy. *N Engl J Med* 1993;**328:**861–868.

68. Stevenson D, Walther F, Long W et al. Controlled trial of a single dose of synthetic surfactant at birth in premature infants weighing 500 to 600 grams. *J Pediatr* 1992;**120:**S3–12.

69. Ferrara TB, Hoekstra RE, Couser RJ et al. Effects of surfactant therapy on outcome of infants with birth weights of 600 to 750 grams. *J Pediatr* 1991;**119:**455–457.

70. Ferrara TB, Hoekstra RE, Couser RJ et al. Survival and follow-up of infants born at 23 to 26 weeks of gestational age: effects of surfactant therapy. *J Pediatr* 1994;**124:**119–124.

71. Schwartz RM, Luby AM, Scanlon JW and Kellogg RJ. Effect of surfactant on morbidity, mortality, and resource use in newborn infants weighing 500 to 1500 g. *N Engl J Med* 1994;**330:**1476–1480.

72. Jobe AH, Mitchell BR and Gunkel JH. Beneficial effects of the combined use of prenatal corticosteroids and postnatal surfactant on preterm infants. *Am J Obstet Gynecol* 1993;**168:**508–513.

73. Leonard CH, Clyman RI, Riecuch RE, Juster RP, Ballard RA and Behle MB. Effect of medical and social risk factors on outcome of prematurity and very low birth weight. *J Pediatr* 1990;**116:**620–626.

74. Resnick MB, Stralka K, Carter RL et al. Effects of birth weight and sociodemographic variables on mental development of neonatal intensive care unit survivors. *Am J Obstet Gynecol* 1990;**162:**374–378.

75. Msall ME, Buck GM, Rogers BT, Merke D, Catanzaro NL and Zorn WA. Risk factors for major neurodevelopmental impairments and need for special education resources in extremely premature infants. *J Pediatr* 1991;**119:**606–614.

76. Ramey CY, Bryant DM, Wasik BH, Sparling JJ, Fendt KH and LaVange LM. Infant health and development program for low birth weight, premature infants: program elements, family participation, and child intelligence. *Pediatrics* 1992;**89:**454–465.

77. Haywood JL, Goldenberg RL, Bronstein J, Nelson KG and Carlo WA. Comparison of perceived and actual rates of survival and freedom from handicap in premature infants. *Am J Obstet Gynecol* 1994;**171:**432–439.

78. de Garis C, Kuhse H, Singer P and Yu VYH. Attitudes of Australian neonatal paediatricians to the treatment of extremely preterm infants. *Aust Paediatr J* 1987;**23**:223–226.
79. Yu VYH. The extremely low birthweight infant: an ethical approach to treatment. *Aust Paediatr J* 1987;**23**:97–103.
80. Young EWD and Stevenson DK. Limiting treatment for extremely premature low-birth-weight infants (500 to 750 g). *Am J Dis Child* 1990;**144**:549–552.
81. Lantos JD, Tyson JE, Allen A et al. Withholding and withdrawing life sustaining treatment in neonatal intensive care: issues for the 1990s. *Arch Dis Child* 1994;**71**:F218–223.
82. Roberton NRC. Should we look after babies less than 800 g? *Arch Dis Child* 1993;**68**:326–329.
83. Yu VYH. Selective non-treatment of newborn infants. *Med J Aust* 1994;**161**:627–629.
84. Victorian Infant Collaborative Study Group. The cost of improving the outcome for infants of birthweight 500 to 999 g in Victoria. *J Paediatr Child Health* 1993;**29**:56–62.
85. Boyle MH, Torrance GW, Sinclair JC and Horwood SP. Economic evaluation of neonatal intensive care of very low birth weight infants. *N Engl J Med* 1983;**308**:1330–1337.
86. Torrance GW and Zipursky A. Cost-effectiveness of antepartum prevention of Rh immunization. *Clin Perinatol* 1984;**11**:267–281.
87. Saigal S, Feeny D, Furlong W, Rosenbaum P, Burrows E and Torrance G. Comparison of the health-related quality of life of extremely low birth weight children and a reference group of children at age eight years. *J Pediatr* 1994;**125**:418–425.

6

Treating Pain in the Neonate

Hans-Ulrich Bucher and
Annemarie Bucher-Schmid

INTRODUCTION

Pain in the newborn infant has until recently been a subject neglected by both clinicians and researchers. Although neonatal nurses have been aware for a long time that even tiny preterm infants react to painful procedures, several misconceptions about pain in newborn infants prevailed until the 1980s:

1. The anatomical structures to receive, transmit and interpret painful stimuli were thought to function only after birth.
2. The observation that preterm infants show weak reaction was misinterpreted as a reduced pain perception.
3. Newborn infants were thought to lack memory, and therefore even if they did feel pain they would not remember it.
4. There was reluctance to use analgesics for fear of severe side effects such as respiratory depression.

Consequently pain in neonates was undertreated and infants were operated on with minimal or no analgesia. In the late 1980s the work of a few pioneers, reviewed in several excellent articles, induced a change in this attitude[1-6], but changes in clinical practice have been slow and efforts for research in this area have remained modest[7,8]. A MEDLINE search for 'pain' and 'newborn' in major subject headings generated only 17 original contributions and 13 reviews or editorials in the 4 year period 1991–1994.

Definition of Pain

The International Association of the Study of Pain defines pain as 'an unpleasant sensory and emotional experience associated with actual or potential tissue damage, or described in terms of such damage'[9]. This definition involves an emotional component that cannot be expressed by preverbal infants. Strictly speaking, pain as a central phenomenon cannot be assessed in newborn infants and therefore nociception is a better term[1]. Nociception is the perception of injury or painful stimuli by nerve endings, spinal tract, midbrain and cortex and does not involve the affective or evaluative component of pain. In this chapter 'pain' will be used in the restricted sense of 'nociception'.

Anatomical and Neurochemical Basis of Pain

Mechanisms of pain perception, modulation and integration are complex in the adult human subject. In the fetus and newborn development makes understanding of these mechanisms even more difficult.

Fitzgerald and Anand give an excellent review on the actual state of knowledge, based mainly on experiments with rats with only a few studies in the human fetus and newborn[10]. They propose a classification of pain based on time course: acute pain (immediate response within seconds and minutes), medium term pain (response within hours and days) and long term pain (lasting for weeks and months).

In this chapter we shall focus on acute pain, which is easier to assess in the newborn infant than is longer term pain.

The easiest way to understand pain transmission in the nervous system is to start with the classical three neurone model established for adult subjects (Figure 6.1). Two types of nerve endings in the skin and inner organs are involved in different qualities of pain perception: type Aδ fibres transmit sharp, localized, pricking pain with rapid onset. C fibres transmit dull, aching, poorly localized pain with slow onset. From the spinal level the pain message travels through several tracts to the midbrain and to the thalamus, from where there are multiple connections to the sensory cortex and limbic system. These pathways are by no means fixed structures but are main lines in a complex neuronal network that undergoes continuous adaptation. It has been demonstrated that connections grow and wane, making the whole system extremely flexible[11].

Figure 6.1 shows only afferent pathways. These must be completed

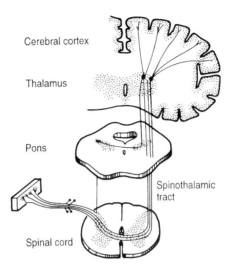

Figure 6.1 Anatomical pathway for pain transmission. Nociceptors in the skin transmit a potentially painful stimulus by slow unmyelinated C fibres or faster thinly myelinated Aδ fibres to the dorsal spinal horn. The majority of the second axons cross by the anterior commissure and reach the thalamus by contralateral tracts; a minority ascend through ipsilateral tracts. The thalamus is connected to the somatosensory areas of the cerebral cortex and to the limbic system.

by descending pathways inhibiting or enhancing potentially painful afferent stimuli at supraspinal and spinal levels.

Numerous neurotransmitters have been suggested as being involved in regulation of pain transmission; they include dopamine, serotonin, substance P and endogenous opioids[11].

Development of Pain Mechanisms

Assessment and treatment of pain in newborn infants, particularly in those born prematurely, are complicated by the dynamics of maturation of specific structures and functions. The milestones in the development of the anatomical structures for pain perception and for the motor response to noxious stimuli are illustrated in Figure 6.2. The basic elements are in place in the first half of gestation. However, there may be considerable delay between formation and function of some structures. Fitzgerald points out that C fibres grow from nociceptors in the skin to the dorsal horn at 22 weeks of gestation but synapses to the ascending neurone are established only

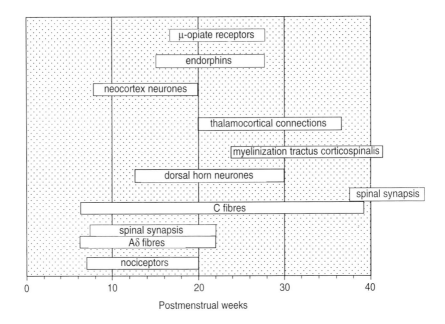

Figure 6.2 Development of nociceptive functions and their anatomical and physiological basis. (Adapted from Anand and Hickey[1] with permission.)

after 40 gestational weeks[12]. Consequently, in the fetus and the infant born before term, noxious stimuli are only propagated through Aδ fibres. This may indicate that preterm infants do not feel dull pain with slow onset but only acute pain.

Maturation of neuronal connections is not a steady and irreversible process. Fitzgerald has shown that the cutaneous receptive fields of dorsal horn cells are large in the newborn rat (corresponding approximately to 24 weeks of human gestation) and gradually diminish over the first two postnatal weeks[13]. These structural changes are consistent with the exaggerated cutaneous reflexes observed in the preterm infant, decreasing towards term[14].

Development of pain mechanisms is a dynamic process. It has been postulated that this development may be affected by excessive noxious stimuli due to invasive clinical procedures[10]. However, exact knowledge of how this may occur and how it could be prevented is lacking.

ASSESSMENT OF PAIN

Successful pain management requires both recognition of pain and correct assessment of pain. One of the reasons for traditional under-treatment of pain in preterm infants is the observation that these immature infants react poorly to a painful stimulus. In clinical practice pain has to be assessed continuously to monitor the effectiveness of a specific treatment. Quantification of pain is fundamental for clinical trials comparing different strategies for pain management.

An ideal method for pain assessment should be easy to apply, reliable and allow quantification for both intensity and duration[15]. A variety of methods have been used but few have been properly evaluated. One of the problems in evaluating single methods is the lack of a gold standard. Most methods have been applied for acute pain caused by interventions producing tissue damage. Attempts to measure chronic pain and long term consequences of acute pain are only beginning[16].

Methods for pain assessment in preverbal infants fall into three categories: physiological, behavioural and hormonal.

Physiological Variables

The most widely used single variable for pain measurement is heart rate, which can be assessed easily and continuously with an electro-cardiograph. An increase in heart rate is usually considered as indicative of pain. The difference in heart rate and the duration of the increase were suggested to correlate with intensity of pain[17]. However, this view has been challenged. Johnston and Strada reported an initial drop in heart rate within the first 6 seconds after a subcutaneous injection followed by a sharp increase in 9 of 14 infants[18]. McIntosh and collaborators found a significant increase in heart rate variability in 35 preterm infants when heel prick was compared with a dummy procedure[19].

Other physiological variables proposed include blood pressure, respiratory rate, transcutaneous PO_2 and PCO_2, arterial oxygen saturation measured by pulse oximetry, sweating, intracranial pressure and cerebral blood volume. Variations in these variables are not specific for pain and show large interindividual differences (Figure 6.3).

The cutaneous flexor reflex is interesting because it is a spinal reflex. It has been used to measure thresholds in preterm infants, which were found to be lower than in term newborns and much lower than in adults[20].

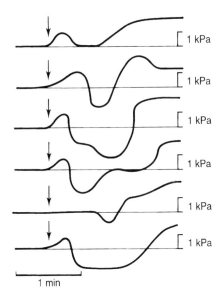

Figure 6.3 Recordings of transcutaneous PO_2 in six preterm infants (gestational age 32–34 weeks, postnatal age 2–4 weeks) during heel prick done under standardized conditions. Note the large interindividual variability, which makes quantification difficult.

Behavioural Variables

Crying, grimacing and body movements are generally known to indicate pain. The problem is to differentiate between distress and other causes. Grunau and collaborators demonstrated that a cluster of facial actions, comprising brow bulging, eyes squeezed shut, deepening of the nasolabial furrow and open mouth, distinguish between invasive and non-invasive procedures[21]. They also analysed spectrograms of cry and defined criteria discriminating pain from non-pain cries.

The most promising approaches for behavioural assessment of pain in newborn infants are coding systems combining several indices. The team of Ruth Grunau and Kenneth Craig in Vancouver developed and evaluated a neonatal facial coding system with nine discrete variables (Table 6.1)[22,23] and an infant body coding system with six discrete variables (Table 6.2)[24]. They found an interobserver reliability of 0.89 and 0.83, respectively. These two scores were used to assess the effect of acute painful interventions. Another scoring

Table 6.1 Neonatal facial coding system

Action	Description
Brow bulge	Bulging, creasing and vertical furrows above and between brows occurring as a result of the lowering and drawing together of the eyebrows
Eye squeeze	Identified by the squeezing or bulging of the eyelids. Bulging of the fatty pads about the infant's eyes is pronounced
Nasolabial furrow	Primarily manifested by the pulling upwards and deepening of the nasolabial furrow (a line or wrinkle which begins adjacent to the nostril wings and runs down and outwards beyond the lip corners)
Open lips	Any separation of the lips is scored as open lips
Stretch mouth (vertical)	Characterized by a tautness at the lip corners coupled with a pronounced downward pull on the jaw. Often stretch mouth is seen when an already wide open mouth is opened a fraction further by an extra pull at the jaw
Stretch mouth (horizontal)	This appears as a distinct horizontal pull at the corners of the mouth
Lip purse	The lips appear as if an 'oo' sound is being pronounced
Taut tongue	Characterized by a raised cupped tongue with sharp tensed edges. The first occurrence of taut tongue is usually easy to see, often occurring with a wide open mouth. After this first occurrence, the mouth may close slightly. Taut tongue is still scorable on the basis of the still visible tongue edges
Chin quiver	An obvious high frequency up–down motion of the lower jaw

Each action is scored as either present or absent, giving a maximal total score of 9.
From Grunau et al[21] with permission.

system was proposed for the measurement of postoperative pain (Table 6.3)[25]. The reliability and clinical validity of this system remains to be demonstrated.

Hormonal Variables

Various hormonal changes have been demonstrated during intensive care and surgical procedures, such as ligation of ductus and cardiac surgery[15,26–28]. The changes included release of catecholamines, steroids, growth hormone and glucagon and suppression of insulin secretion. These responses resulted in the breakdown of carbo-

Table 6.2 Infant body coding system

Action	Description
Hand/foot movements	Include flexion, extension or rotation at the wrist, and spreading, grasping, or twitching of the fingers. Foot movements include flexion, extension or rotation at the ankle and spreading, twitching or flaring of the toes
Arm movements	Include well modulated, jerky and/or limited movements, and well modulated movements that involve a transition from flexion to extension, or vice versa, or ad/abduction accomplished smoothly without jerkiness. In well modulated movements the arc of motion appears controlled and unrestricted with one movement frequently moving into the next. Jerky arm movements involve sudden abrupt oscillation from extension to flexion, or vice versa, dramatic startles, and twitches, or movements that are restricted by something in their path. Limited movements included twisting, or writhing of the limbs close to the body
Leg movements	Include well modulated, jerky and/or limited movements. The descriptions of these above apply here
Head movements	Include lateral activity, head turn, and neck flexion or extension
Torso movements	Include resisting, arching, twisting or writhing in the torso

Each action is scored as either present or absent, giving a maximum total score of 6.
From Craig et al[24] with permission.

hydrate, protein and fat stores with prolonged hyperglycaemia and increase of lactate, total ketone bodies, non-esterified fatty acids and amino acids and an elevated nitrogen excretion.

The difference in hormone levels can be used to quantify stress response, as shown by Anand and colleagues in their landmark study on the effects of fentanyl in preterm infants undergoing surgical ligation of a patent ductus arteriosus[29]. The drawbacks of the assessment of the hormonal response to pain are: (1) that blood samples have to be taken, which might favour iatrogenic anaemia, especially in small preterm infants; (2) that expert laboratory facilities are required; and (3) that the result is only available later and too late to correct inadequate therapy.

Which Method for Assessment of Pain Should be Chosen?

None of the available methods for assessment of pain in the newborn infant, who cannot communicate verbally, is ideal. With the excep-

Table 6.3 Postoperative pain score

Behaviour	0 (poor)	1 (mediocre)	2 (satisfactory)
Sleep during preceding hour	None	Short naps between 5 and 10 minutes	Longer naps >10 minutes
Facial expression of pain	Marked, constant	Less marked, intermittent	Calm, relaxed
Quality of cry	Screaming, painful, high-pitched	Modulated (can be distracted by normal sound)	No cry
Spontaneous motor activity	Thrashing around, incessant agitation	Moderate agitation	Normal
Spontaneous excitability and responsiveness to ambient stimulation	Tremulous, clonic movements, spontaneous Moro reflexes	Excessive reactivity (to any stimulation)	Quiet
Flexion of fingers and toes	Very pronounced, marked and constant	Less marked, intermittent	Absent
Sucking	Absent or disorganized	Intermittent (three or four) and stops with crying	Strong, rhythmic with pacifying effect
Global evaluation of tone	Strong hypertonicity	Moderate hypertonicity	Normal for age
Consolability	None after 2 minutes	Quiet after 1 minute of effort	Calm before 1 minute
Sociability (eye contact) response to voice, smile, real interest in face	Absent	Difficult to obtain	Easy and prolonged

Infants with a total score of 15–20 have arbitrarily been considered to have adequate postoperative pain management. From Bell[9] with permission; adapted from Barrier G et al[25].

tion of the flexor withdrawal response, all responses depend on appropriate function of the pain pathways from the nociceptor to the cortex, which undergoes modification by inhibiting and enhancing stimuli at spinal, thalamic and cortical levels. The response is further dependent on the range of a measured or observed parameter, which may differ considerably in the same infants at different times and between individuals. Therefore several important influences affecting both the sensitivity and specificity of single indicators must be considered.

For clinical situations physiological and behavioural variables give an immediate feedback for the nurses and doctors executing painful procedures. For scientific purposes a combination of several variables, preferably from different categories, increases the validity of pain assessment. Finally, the duration of the painful episode has to be taken into account. For short term distress, monitoring behavioural and physiological variables is preferable, whereas for pain lasting for hours and even days measuring plasma changes of hormone levels and the metabolic consequences may be more relevant.

PREVENTION OF DISTRESS AND PAIN IN NEONATAL INTENSIVE CARE

Prevention is superior to treatment. This medical axiom is also valid for distress and pain in newborn infants. As most pain in neonates is iatrogenic, e.g. the result of specific diagnostic and therapeutic procedures, reflections on how to reduce or avoid pain are most important.

Several strategies for preventing or minimizing pain in the critically ill neonate have been proposed (Table 6.4)[9,30]. The recent technical advances in non-invasive monitoring, especially of blood gases, have contributed considerably to reaching this goal. Strong indication for blood samples, taking a minimal amount of blood, and clustering of painful procedures so that the baby can recover for longer periods are steps in the same direction. Very often the intensity and duration of pain can be reduced by skilled and efficient execution of invasive procedures.

Table 6.4 Strategies to prevent or minimize stress in the neonate

- Use non-invasive monitoring devices
- Reduce noise (close incubator doors gently)
- Protect from light (shade infant's eyes)
- Cluster blood drawings by heel lance or venepuncture
- Establish central vessel access to minimize vein and artery punctures
- Have only expert staff attempt potentially painful procedures
- Replace tape by self adhesive bandage
- Do intratracheal suctioning only if indicated
- Ensure proper premedication before invasive procedures

Modified from NAACOG Committee on Practice. *OGN Nursing Practice Resource: Prevention, Recognition, and Management of Neonatal Pain.* Washington, DC: NAACOG, 1991.

TREATMENT OF PAIN

A rational approach to the selection of the appropriate treatment in a particular situation should be based, on the one hand, on evaluation of the localization, intensity and duration of the noxious stimulus. On the other hand, evidence of the efficacy of pharmacological and non-pharmacological methods for pain relief should be available. The selection of an analgesic drug should include the following information:

1. Optimal therapeutic serum concentration, e.g. range between minimal analgesic serum concentration and lowest serum concentration at which severe side effects have been observed.
2. The pharmacokinetics of the candidate drug and its metabolites and the factors affecting metabolism and elimination.
3. Effects other than analgesia, such as respiratory depression, that may be more or less desired.

There are important differences between neonates and older children or adults and information available from studies in older patients cannot simply be extrapolated to neonates, especially when they are born well before term.

This section draws together the scarce data from neonatal studies but the reader must be aware that much of the information is preliminary and has to be confirmed in the future.

Effectiveness of Pain Management

The first question we should answer before choosing a particular method for pain treatment is: what is the evidence for its effectiveness? This should be based on a prospectively designed controlled clinical trial, preferably a randomized, placebo controlled, masked trial.

Table 6.5 gives an overview of specific interventions for pain that have been tested in a clinical trial and that we could identify with a MEDLINE literature search. Compared with other treatments in newborn infants, such as surfactant administration or closure of ductus arteriosus with indomethacin, this number is small. This may be due to problems with the design of such trials (for example defining outcome variables), a selective rejection for publication of trials with negative results, or a lack of interest in performing such trials[28,29,31-43].

The number of patients recruited in these trials is generally small and therefore only large differences can be expected to be demonstrated.

Table 6.5 Review of controlled trials for pain treatment in neonates

Design	Cause of pain	Patients' characteristics	n	Controls	Intervention	Outcome measurement	Experimental group	Control group	P	Reference
	Heel prick	Healthy term infants, 5–6 days	18	18	Mechanical lancet (Autolet)	Palmar water loss (g m^{-2} h^{-1})	37.3 (27–114)	60.7 (18–85)	<0.005	[31]
db, pc	Heel prick	Term infants, 28–54 hours	12	12	3 ml sucrose 12%, 2 min before prick	Relative crying time (%)	42	80	<0.001	[32]
db, pc	Heel prick	Healthy term infants	26	26	Sucrose 7.5%	Relative crying time (%)	74.30	73.20	NS	[33]
db, pc	Heel prick	Healthy term infants, 3–6 days	26	26	12.5 mg lignocaine ointment	Behaviour scale / Increase in heart rate 10 min after prick	3.8 / 22	4.9 / 16	<0.05 / NS	[35]
db, pc	Heel prick	34–41 gestational weeks, 4–11 days	15	15	5% lignocaine ointment 1 h before prick	Behaviour score: median (range)	5 (1 to 5)	5 (2 to 5)	NS	[34]
	Heel prick	26–34 gestational weeks, 7–35 days, incubator care	35	Same infants	EMLA cream 1 h before prick / Spring loaded device (Glucolet) / Tactile and vocal stimulation by nurse	Heart rate, respiratory rate, tcPO_2, tcPCO_2	No effect on absolute heart rate, tcPO_2 and tcPCO_2 / Decrease in heart rate variability after glucolet and comfort / Increase in heart rate variability after EMLA cream			[36]
db, pc	Heel prick	27–34 gestational weeks, 10–67 days, 900–1900 g, intermediate care	16	Same infants	2 ml sucrose 50% orally 2 min before prick	Heart rate (increase from baseline in bpm) / Relative crying time (%)	34.4 (SD 13.5) / 67.0 (SD 28.1)	49.4 (14.1) / 88.6 (14.2)	0.005 / 0.002	[44]
	Lumbar puncture	Newborn infants <4 weeks	38	39	Local anaesthesia: 0.1 ml kg^{-1} 1% lignocaine	Heart rate (bpm) / Minimum tcPO_2 (mmHg)	146.4 (SEM 3.1) / 46.9 (SEM 4.9)	148.5 (SEM 3.1) / 46.8 (SEM 4.9)	0.64 / 0.98	[41]
db, pc	Circumcision	Normal term boys	20	20	Dorsal penile nerve blockade with 1% lignocaine	Relative crying time (%) / Cortisol serum concentration (nmol l^{-1})	23 (SEM 7.6) / 386 (SEM 36)	68 (SEM 7.8) / 532 (SEM 44)	<0.001 / <0.05	[37]
db, pc	Circumcision	Term infants, 28–54 hours	10	10	Sucrose 12% / Sucrose 12% and pacifier	Crying time (%) / Crying time (%)	49 / 31	67 / 67	<0.05 / <0.01	[32]
	Circumcision	Term boys	20 / 20 / 20 / 20	21 / 21 / 21 / 21	Classical music / Intrauterine sounds / Classical music and pacifier / Intrauterine sounds and pacifier	Blood pressure, / Transcutaneous PO_2, / Heart rate, / Behavioural assessment scale	No consistent effect / No consistent effect / No consistent effect / No consistent effect	— / — / — / —	— / — / — / —	[42]

Design	Procedure	Population	n	n	Intervention	Outcome	Treatment	Control	p	Ref
db, pc	Circumcision	Healthy term boys, ≥2500 g	15	14	Topical 30% lidocaine cream	β-endorphin after circumcision	65 (SD 57)	114 (SD 54)	0.02	[43]
db, pc	Circumcision	Healthy term boys	23	21	Paracetamol (Tylenol) 15 mg kg^{-1} per dose every 6 h	Increase in crying time (%)	7 (SD 18)	15 (SD 20)	NS	[38]
						Comfort score 2 h after circumcision	2.56	2.64	NS	
						Heart rate (increase from baseline in bpm)	29.6 (SD 21.8)	22.3 (SD 19.4)	NS	
db, pc	Mechanical ventilation, administration of surfactant	Preterm infants <34 weeks gestation with respiratory distress syndrome	21	20	Continuous morphine (loading dose: 200 µg kg^{-1}, maintenance dose: 25 µg kg^{-1} h^{-1})	Crying time (%)	0.64 (SD 0.34)	0.49 (SD 0.46)	NS	[28]
						Adrenaline at 24 h (nmol l^{-1})	0.69 (IQR 0.36 to 1.34)	1.34 (IQR 0.69 to 2.19)	<0.001	
						Noradrenaline at 24 h (nmol l^{-1})	2.89 (IQR 1.32 to 9.27)	4.87 (IQR 3.03 to 11.64)	<0.01	
						Heart rate (change during first 6 h in bpm)	−5 (IQR −17.5 to 5)	−5 (IQR −10 to 5)	NS	
						Blood pressure (change during first 6 h in mmHg)	−4 (IQR −8 to 0)	1 (IQR −5 to 7)	NS	
db, pc	Intratracheal suctioning and other intensive care procedures	Newborn infants 670–4260 g, 25–41 gestational weeks, mechanically ventilated	42	42	Pethidine 1 mg kg^{-1} 15 min before procedure	β-endorphin 2 h after procedure (pg ml^{-1})	57.6 (CI 10.3 to 426.0)	68.2 (CI 10.3 to 230.0)	NS	[39]
						Cortisol 2 h after procedure (nmol l^{-1})	325 (CI 60 to 3050)	330 (CI 60 to 4450)	NS	
						Duration of hypoxaemia (s)	36 (CI 20 to 53)	82 (CI 46 to 117)	<0.001	
						Behavioural score (max. 12)	5	7.7	< 0.01	
db, pc	Ligation of patent ductus arteriosus	Preterm infants	8	8	Fentanyl	Adrenaline, noradrenaline, urinary 3-methylhistidine:creatine ratio				[29]
						Postoperative complications				
db, pc	Cardiac surgery	Mean gestational age 40 weeks, mean weight 3.6 kg	30	15	Sufentanil (3 doses 5–10 µg kg^{-1} iv) Postop sufentanil (2–4 µg kg^{-1} h^{-1} iv) or fentanyl (8-15 µg kg^{-1} h^{-1} iv)	Perioperative change in adrenaline (nmol l^{-1})	1.8 (SEM 1.6)	6.2 (SEM 2.4)	<0.025	[40]
						Increase in lactate (mmol l^{-1})	3.9 (SEM 0.4)	6.8 (SEM 1.4)	<0.025	
						Postoperative death	0/30	4/15	0.009	

db, double blind (masked); pc, placebo controlled; values are mean (range); CI, 95% confidence interval; IQR, interquartile range; SD, standard deviation; SEM, standard error of mean; tc, transcutaneous; NS, not significant.

The best investigated model for acute pain is heel prick but this model poses methodological problems because changes in outcome variables due to warming, cleaning and squeezing the heel, which are not considered to be painful, cannot be differentiated from those due to the heel stab. McIntosh et al found no difference between a heel prick and a dummy procedure (which included all elements of the procedure except heel prick) in the absolute change of heart rate, respiratory rate, transcutaneous PO_2 and PCO_2 but did find a significant difference in the variability of these variables[19]. The effect of confounding factors can be minimized by a careful design with an identical detailed protocol for the experimental and the control procedure. The effects of a mechanical lancet, a pacifier, sucrose and local anaesthesia have been investigated with the heel prick model with controversial results, which will be commented on later.

Several methods for relief of pain during and after circumcision have been tested. Whereas local anaesthesia[43], dorsal penile nerve blockade[37] and sucrose[32] given immediately before the procedure had significant effect on stress response , classical music and intrauterine sounds[42] did not. The use of a pacifier had a calming effect additional to the gustatory stimulation with sucrose[32], but it had no consistent effect in combination with acoustic stimulation[42]. These results can be criticized because the outcome variables based on physiological changes and behaviour are not specific.

One study investigating the effect of local anaesthesia before lumbar puncture showed no benefit[41]. Destabilization of physiological parameters was more influenced by the preparatory procedures than by the lumbar puncture itself and these were more prolonged in the group with local anaesthesia.

Two studies have shown a significant reduction in hormonal stress response by continuous infusion of morphine or fentanyl in mechanically ventilated newborn infants[27,28]. This effect was not seen if infants were only paralysed with pancuronium without systemic analgesia. In a similar patient group pethidine administered 15 minutes before intratracheal suctioning or other painful procedure had no significant effect on β-endorphin and cortisol in the serum but had a favourable effect on the duration of hypoxaemia and the behavioural score[39].

Two studies by Anand and coworkers demonstrated a profound effect of fentanyl and sufentanil in addition to conventional anaesthesia on hormonal and metabolic response in newborn infants during cardiac surgery[29,40]. These authors also found reduced complications and fewer deaths in the deep analgesia group. Although these studies have been criticized for their methodology, their relevance for the effectiveness of analgesia in newborn infants during major surgery cannot be denied.

Non-pharmacological Pain Management

Non-pharmacological methods, as described above (see Table 6.4), are easy to apply, inexpensive and well accepted by nurses and parents, and therefore should be integrated into the basic care of sick newborn infants. Only a pacifier, classical music, intrauterine sounds and comforting by a nurse have been formally tested, with ambiguous results (Table 6.5). An interesting observation, implying that the mechanism does not involve supraspinal levels, was the positive effect of contralateral counterirritation, e.g. massage of the opposite leg, during heel prick[30]. The effectiveness of massage procedures for newborns remains to be demonstrated. Non-pharmacological methods can be combined and this may increase their effect but these methods do not seem to be sufficient to relieve acute pain from noxious procedures and they should not prevent the use of more potent analgesics.

Sucrose

There has recently been special interest in the use of sucrose and its mechanisms of action. Blass and Hoffmeyer found that the calming effect of sucrose in rat pups could be fully eliminated by pretreatment with naltrexone, an opiate antagonist[32]. They concluded that sucrose acts by stimulating the release of endogenous opiates. There are three clinical trials investigating the effect of sucrose on crying during a heel prick (Table 6.5); two show a significant reduction of the relative time the infant spent crying during the procedure[32,44] and one did not[33]. The differences in design, gestational age and dose of sucrose can hardly explain this discrepancy. It is more likely that the effect is relatively small and the behavioural response is influenced by gestational age, initial behavioural state and other factors. As with any other drug, sucrose has potential side effects that may be relevant in very immature infants, such as hyperglycaemia, fluid overload, increased risk of necrotizing enterocolitis due to its high osmolarity and detrimental effects in the rare fructose intolerance[44]. In infants above 34 weeks gestational age sucrose given immediately before a heel prick is likely to do more good than harm.

Local Anaesthesia and Peripheral Nerve Blockade

Reversible block of pain pathways at receptor, peripheral nerve or spinal level has the benefit of few systemic side effects and there-fore it seems to be appropriate for localized procedure related pain. Three clinical studies, however, investigating the effect of topical lignocaine (lidocaine *USP*) ointment on pain response to heel prick, showed a reduced response in only a few of the parameters tested (Table 6.5)[34-36]. In another trial, local injection of lignocaine before lumbar puncture showed no effect[41]. In contrast, two trials during circumcision have demonstrated a significant effect of topi-cal ointment with lignocaine and of dorsal penile nerve blockade[37,43]. We conclude from these controversial results that more studies focused on the method of application and the dose are needed.

One step in this direction is an in vitro study that investigated the feasibility of percutaneous application of lignocaine in preterm infants[45]. It was demonstrated that there is a strong inverse correlation between gestational age and skin permeability, and it was calculated that the risk of toxicity for systemic absorption is negligible, even for very immature infants.

The choice of local anaesthetics for neonates is limited. Prilocaine, which is one component of the popular EMLA cream used in infants over 1 year old, is not recommended for neonates because it may induce methaemoglobinaemia in preterm infants who have reduced methaemoglobin reductase activity[46]. Lignocaine is therefore pre-ferred. The technical aspects of peripheral nerve blockade have recently been reviewed by Yaster et al[47].

In a randomized controlled clinical trial, spinal anaesthesia has been shown to reduce the risk for apnoea in former preterm infants undergoing herniotomy[48].

Non-steroidal Analgesics

These drugs also have an anti-inflammatory and antipyretic effect[49]. The specific mechanism through which they produce analgesia is not known.

Paracetamol

Paracetamol (acetaminophen *USP*) is probably the most widely used analgesic drug in infants and children beyond the neonatal period. The only trial of its effectiveness in newborn infants that we could find failed to demonstrate an effect on behaviour, heart rate and crying time during and after circumcision. It has a relatively weak analgesic effect that is difficult to assess in neonates, but may be indicated for its antipyretic action. The optimal serum concentration is quoted[50] as 15–20 mg ml[-1]. Liver toxicity is likely if serum concentration exceeds 120 mg ml[-1] 4 hours after ingestion[51]. One pharmacokinetic study found serum elimination half life of 2.8 hours (95% confidence interval 1.2 to 4.4 hours) for neonates, comparable with that of older infants and children[50]. These authors cite two cases of grossly prolonged serum half lives of up to 26 hours after overdose. They also found prolonged and less predictable elimination after rectal application. An oral dose of 15–20 mg kg[-1] paracetamol, resulting in peak serum concentration of 10–20 mg ml[-1], can be considered both effective and safe in term infants beyond the first week of life. Accumulation can be avoided with minimum intervals of 6 hours.

Acetylsalicylic acid
Acetylsalicylic acid (aspirin) should not be given to neonates, for it may inhibit platelet aggregation and increase the risk of bleeding[52]. It also may be associated with the Reye syndrome in combination with a viral infection[53].

Indomethacin
Indomethacin is used in adults and children for rheumatic pain. Due to its strong prostaglandin synthetase inhibiting action it is administered to preterm infants for closure of a patent ductus arteriosus. Despite numerous clinical studies its analgesic effect has not been documented in newborn infants. Given the well known renal and gastrointestinal side effects it cannot be recommended for pain relief in newborn infants. However, when indomethacin is indicated for closure of the ductus arteriosus reduction of other analgesics may be possible.

Opioids
Opioids are the most potent analgesics for adults and children as well as for neonates; however, there are several peculiarities that have to be taken into account when newborn infants are given opioids.

The oldest and best investigated opioid in neonates is morphine, which will be the standard for the following consideration. The newer opioids such as pethidine (meperidine *USP*), fentanyl and other derivatives will be compared with morphine.

Pharmacokinetics

Pharmacokinetic studies after single bolus injection and with continuous infusion showed reduced clearance, greater volume of distribution and prolonged elimination half life of between 2.3 and 28 hours in newborn infants, compared with 2–3 hours in adults (Table 6.6)[54-62]. Factors responsible for this prolongation and large variation in elimination may be slow metabolism in the liver[63] and reduced renal clearance.

Pharmacokinetics may change rapidly with age. For sulfentanil Greely et al in three infants found a reduction of elimination half life from a mean of 653 minutes in week 1 to 217 minutes in week 4 – a reduction of 66%[59].

A specific problem in newborn infants during their first days of life is intrauterine exposure to opioids. Infants of drug dependent mothers may not only show withdrawal symptoms but may also be less sensitive to the analgesic effect of opioids. As opioids are frequently given to mothers to relieve pain during delivery, their infants may receive significant quantities across the placenta. Serum concentrations have been shown to increase up to 4 days after birth. This preload has to be taken into account when starting opioids in the first days of life.

Optimal serum concentration

The minimum serum concentration for morphine associated with suppression of clinical signs of pain during surgery in infants and children was found[64] to range between 43 and 86 ng ml^{-1}. It has been suggested that the minimal analgesic concentration may increase with lower gestational age and with reduced number of specific receptors[30]. This need for a higher concentration may be compensated for by superior diffusion across the blood–brain barrier and a lower fraction of protein binding (20% in neonates versus 30% in adults), leaving a larger fraction of free serum opioids. Further studies are required to define the relative contribution of each factor in lowering or increasing the minimal effective serum concentration.

To fix an upper limit for a safe serum concentration is virtually impossible because convulsions probably related to morphine have been reported with relatively low concentrations of 61 and 90 ng ml^{-1} and because side effects such as respiratory depression correlate with serum concentrations already in the proposed therapeutic range[65]. Chay et al suggested an optimal serum concentration of 125 ng ml^{-1} (95% confidence interval 116 to 135 ng ml^{-1}) based on a study of 19 neonates, both preterm and term[56].

Table 6.6 Pharmacokinetic studies on opioids

Drug	Patients				Indication for analgesia	Type of study	Plasma steady state concentration (ng ml⁻¹)	Volume of distribution at steady state (l kg⁻¹)	Clearance (ml min⁻¹ kg⁻¹)	Slow distribution half life T/2a (minutes)	Elimination half life T/2b (hours)	Reference
	n	Gestational age (weeks)	Postnatal age (days)	Weight (kg)								
Morphine	9	24–37	3–12	—	Mechanical ventilation	c: 10–40 µg kg⁻¹ h⁻¹	113 (26–210)		4.7 (0.8–9.6)			[54]
Morphine	10	26–30	2.3 (SD 0.8)	1.02 (SD 0.24)	Mechanical ventilation	s: 0.1 mg kg⁻¹	11.9–154.0	1.84 (SD 0.84)	3.39 (SD 3.28)	50 (SD 35)	10.0 (SD 3.7)	[55]
	7	31–37	1.85 (SD 1.0)	1.87 (SD 0.4)			10.1–108	5.18 (SD 1.6)	9.6 (SD 4.0)	41 (SD 19)	7.4 (SD 1.7)	
	3	38–40	1.3 (SD 0.6)	3.0 (SD 0.2)				2.9 (SD 2.1)	15.5 (SD 10.0)	19 (SD 8)	6.7 (SD 4.6)	
Morphine	12	>36	1–7	2.5–3.6	Cardiac surgery	c: 20 µg kg⁻¹ h⁻¹	45.2 (21.1–68.8)	3.3 (1.7–4.5)	5.5 (3.2–8.4)		7.2 (5.1–15.8)	[57]
Morphine	7	37–41	1–4	2.94–3.6	Mechanical ventilation	c: 7.5–30 µg kg⁻¹ h⁻¹	192 (75–397)	2.07 (0.24–3.34)	2.31 (0.85–3.24)		7.6 (5.8–11)	[56]
	12	32–36	1–3	1.35–3.54	Mechanical ventilation	c: 7.5–30 µg kg⁻¹ h⁻¹	150 (70–420)	2.04 (0.6–3.68)	2.67 (0.51–4.05)		10.6 (5.5–13.4)	
Pethidine	9	36–41	0.3–4.0	2.4–4.5	Surgery, mechanical ventilation	s: 1 mg kg⁻¹		5.6 (3.7–9.2)	7.2 (5.3–13.8)		10.7 (4.9–16.8)	[58]
	6	36–42	26–73	2.3–8.8	Surgery, mechanical ventilation	s: 1 mg kg⁻¹		8.0 (4.9–11.0)	9.7 (4.1–20.5)		8.2 (5.7–31.7)	
	5	28–33	4–65	1.6–2.4	Surgery, mechanical ventilation	s: 1 mg kg⁻¹		8.8 (3.3–9.4)	3.5 (1.8–34.9)		11.9 (3.3–59.4)	
Fentanyl	14	—	—	1.4–4.0	Major surgery	s: 10–50 µg kg⁻¹		5.1 (1.3–13.5)	17.9 (3.4–47.4)		5.3 (1.3–15.9)	[61]
Fentanyl	14	32–40	1–71	1.9–3.9	Surgery	s: 54.1 (SD 2.3) µg kg⁻¹		8.3 (4.8–11.9)	19.2 (0–32.8)		5.4 (3.1–8.3)	[60]
Alfentanil	22	25–36	0–4	0.69–4.084	Mechanical ventilation	s: 20 µg kg⁻¹		0.5 (0.13–1.04)	0.87 (0.4–9.6)	7.6 (2.0–38.1)	5.4 (1.1–20.9)	[62]
	14	25–36	0–4	0.69–4.084	Mechanical ventilation	c: 3 or 5 µg kg⁻¹ h⁻¹*	29 (1–104)					
Sufentanil	3	—	2–7	3.0–3.3	Cardiac surgery	s: 10 µg kg⁻¹		2.7 (2.6–2.9)	4.2 (1.7–6.7)	20.5 (17.7–23.2)	10.6 (5.5–19.0)	[59]
		—	20–28	—	Cardiac surgery	s: 10 µg kg⁻¹		3.4 (3.2–3.6)	17.3 (12.9–19.3)	8.8 (7.1–10.5)	3.6 (2.7–4.1)	

Values are mean (range) or (SD).

s, single bolus; c, constant infusion.

*After 15 or 20 µg kg⁻¹ loading dose.

Physiological effects

Opioids bind predominantly to two of a variety of opioid receptors, to μ1 receptors associated with supraspinal analgesia, and to μ2 receptors associated with spinal analgesia, respiratory depression and gastrointestinal motility. The effect on respiration can be quantified with the ventilatory response to carbon dioxide and has been shown to be dose dependent[66]. The respiratory depression may last longer than the analgesic effect, which was attributed to the persistence of morphine-6-glucuronide metabolized in the liver from morphine[63]. Bronchospasm induced by opioids may also be a problem in mechanically ventilated infants. Reduction of intestinal motility results in delayed gastric emptying, abdominal distension and constipation, all of which may be important side effects in neonates. An increased tone of detrusor muscle of the bladder may cause urinary retention. Hypotension may become significant in dehydrated patients. Morphine has been reported to cause bradycardia with high serum concentration (300 ng ml^{-1}): this was reversible within 2–8 hours[56]. Convulsions are an infrequent but serious complication that can occur at relatively low serum concentration[65].

Physical dependence on opiates may be established after 1–2 weeks. Withdrawal signs are well known in the newborns of drug dependent mothers who have been exposed to opioids for prolonged periods before birth. These signs include agitation, tachypnoea, tachycardia, feeding problems and diarrhoea. Withdrawal can be managed with careful tapering of dosage over several days.

Antagonists

All the effects of opioids, including analgesia, are completely reversible by antagonists, of which naloxone (Narcan) is the most widely used in newborn infants. Naloxone is mainly given to reverse respiratory depression during postnatal adaptation in newborns of mothers given opiates in labour and opiate dependent mothers. The recommended dose is 0.01–0.1 mg kg^{-1}. Higher doses could precipitate withdrawal symptoms in the infants of opiate dependent mothers. As naloxone is rapidly eliminated from serum, its duration of action is much shorter than the agonist it is used to reverse and therefore repetitive administration may be necessary.

Suggestions for dosage

Recommendation for dosage is hardly possible in view of the heterogeneity of the neonatal population and the multitude of factors affecting pharmacokinetics. To cope with this dilemma, Yaster and

Maxwell recommend titration at the bedside[66]. This means continuous assessment of the desired effects and monitoring for undesired effects. Unfortunately no assay is available for routine measurement of serum concentration in small aliquots of blood, which would allow individual dose adjustment. Table 6.7 gives commonly used doses which should be considered as a rough guide.

Table 6.7 Suggested dose for opioids

Opioid	Single i.v. dose	Continuous infusion	Oral dose	Comments
Morphine	0.1 mg kg^{-1}	10–40 µg kg^{-1} h^{-1}	0.3 mg kg^{-1}	Poor intestinal absorption
Pethidine	1.0 mg kg^{-1}	—	1.0 mg kg^{-1}	Good intestinal absorption
Fentanyl	10–50 µg kg^{-1}	Loading dose: 10 µg kg^{-1} Maintenance dose: 2–5 µg kg^{-1} h^{-1}	—	Tolerance may require increase of dose on successive days
Alfentanil	20 µg kg^{-1}	3–5 µg kg^{-1} h^{-1}	—	—
Sufentanil	10 µg kg^{-1}	—	—	—

Pethidine
Pethidine is a synthetic opioid and widely used in neonates. It is ten times less potent than morphine but has very similar effects. Pethidine depresses respiration less than morphine.

Pethidine is much better absorbed from the gastrointestinal tract than morphine, making it the most widely used oral narcotic. Tolerance develops with time, requiring dose escalation.

Fentanyl and derivatives
Fentanyl is a synthetic opioid 100 times more potent than morphine, with rapid onset and brief duration (Table 6.6). It is used for short procedures, such as intratracheal intubation (10 µg kg^{-1}) and for cardiac surgery in higher doses (Table 6.7). Oral transmucosal application of 15–20 µg kg^{-1} fentanyl citrate became popular as the fentanyl 'lollipop' in children but has not yet been tested in neonates[67].

One serious side effect of fentanyl is reduction of pulmonary and thoracic compliance, which may impede ventilation. This can be overcome by combining the drug with muscle relaxants[68].

In contrast to other opioids fentanyl may rapidly induce tolerance, which may result in the need for progressive increases in dose.

Sufentanil is a fentanyl derivative which is ten times more potent than fentanyl. Alfentanil is 3–10 times less potent than fentanyl and has an extremely short duration of action[62]. Both are used for neonates undergoing cardiac surgery[40].

Supplementary Sedative Drugs

Benzodiazepines (diazepam, midazolam) and chloral hydrate are frequently combined with analgesics. They may be useful for treating agitation. Their effectiveness for neonates has not been demonstrated in a randomized, controlled clinical trial. As they do not have an analgesic effect they should not be given alone to relieve pain. Both diazepam and chloral hydrate have long elimination half lives, which increases the risk of intoxication with repeated administration. Midazolam has an elimination half life of 1.2–1.7 hours which makes it first choice for brief rapid sedation[30].

OBJECTIVES FOR FUTURE RESEARCH

The increasing willingness of the medical community to accept that neonates feel pain and therefore need treatment is the result of pioneering research. However, many gaps in our knowledge remain to be filled before rational treatment can be given to the tiniest preterm infant.

Objectives for future research may be:

- Better knowledge of the development of anatomical structures and the neurochemical processes involved in transmitting, integrating and perceiving pain.
- Refinement of methods for assessment of short term and long term pain in preterm infants.
- Randomized controlled clinical trials to evaluate different strategies for reducing pain in newborn infants.
- Definition of optimal serum concentrations for specific analgesics for different gestational ages.
- Evaluation of factors affecting pharmacokinetics and efficacy of specific drugs.
- Development of new drugs with specific analgesic action and minimal undesired effects.
- Application of analgesics with local and systemic action through intact skin or mucous membranes.

Clarification of these and other points should improve management of pain and finally improve long term outcome.

REFERENCES

1. Anand KJ and Hickey PR. Pain and its effects in the human neonate and fetus. *N Engl J Med* 1987;**317:**1321–1329.
2. Colditz PB. Management of pain in the newborn infant. *J Paediatr Child Health* 1991;**27:**11–15.
3. Fitzgerald M and McIntosh N. Pain and analgesia in the newborn. *Arch Dis Child* 1989;**64:**441–443.
4. Porter F. Pain in the newborn. *Clin Perinatol* 1989;**16:**549–564.
5. Schechter NL. The undertreatment of pain in children: an overview. *Pediatr Clin North Am* 1989;**36:**781–794.
6. Schuster A and Lenard HG. Pain in newborns and prematures: current practice and knowledge. *Brain Dev* 1990;**12:**459–465.
7. Fernandez CV and Rees EP. Pain management in Canadian level 3 neonatal intensive care units. *Can Med Assoc J* 1994;**150:**499–504.
8. Bauchner H, May A and Coates E. Use of analgesic agents for invasive medical procedures in pediatric and neonatal intensive care units. *J Pediatr* 1992;**121:**647–649.
9. Bell SG. The neonatal pain management guideline: implications for neonatal intensive care. Agency for Health Care Policy and Research. *Neonatal Netw* 1994;**13:**9–17.
10. Fitzgerald M and Anand KJS. Developmental neuroanatomy and neurophysiology of pain. In: Schechter NL, Berde CB and Yaster M (eds) *Pain in Infants, Children, and Adolescents.* Baltimore: Williams & Wilkins, 1993: 11–31.
11. Anand KJ and Carr DB. The neuroanatomy, neurophysiology, and neurochemistry of pain, stress, and analgesia in newborns and children. *Pediatr Clin North Am* 1989;**36:**795–822.
12. Fitzgerald M. Development of pain mechanisms. *Br Med Bull* 1991;**47:**667–675.
13. Fitzgerald M. The post-natal development of cutaneous afferent fibre input and receptive field organization in the rat dorsal horn. *J Physiol (Lond)* 1985;**364:**1–18.
14. Andrews K and Fitzgerald M. The cutaneous withdrawal reflex in human neonates: sensitization, receptive fields, and the effects of contralateral stimulation. *Pain* 1994;**56:**95–101.
15. Porter F. Pain assessment in children: infants. In: Schechter JL, Berde CB and Yaster M (eds) *Pain in Infants, Children, and Adolescents.* Baltimore: Williams & Wilkins, 1993:87–96.
16. Taddio A, Goldbach M, Ipp M, Stevens B and Koren G. Effect of neonatal circumcision on pain responses during vaccination in boys. *Lancet* 1995;**344:**291–292.
17. Owens ME and Todt EH. Pain in infancy: neonatal reaction to a heel lance. *Pain* 1984;**20:**77–86.
18. Johnston CC and Strada ME. Acute pain response in infants: a multidimensional description. *Pain* 1986;**24:**373–382.

19. McIntosh N, Van Veen L and Brameyer H. The pain of heel prick and its measurement in preterm infants. *Pain* 1993;**52**:71–74.

20. Fitzgerald M, Shaw A and McIntosh N. Postnatal development of the cutaneous flexor reflex: comparative study of preterm infants and newborn rat pups. *Dev Med Child Neurol* 1988;**30**:520–526.

21. Grunau RV, Johnston CC and Craig KD. Neonatal facial and cry responses to invasive and non-invasive procedures. *Pain* 1990;**42**:295–305.

22. Grunau RV and Craig KD. Pain expression in neonates: facial action and cry. *Pain* 1987;**28**:395–410.

23. Craig KD, Hadjistavropoulos HD, Grunau RV and Whitfield MF. A comparison of two measures of facial activity during pain in the newborn child. *J Pediatr Psychol* 1994;**19**:305–318.

24. Craig KD, Whitfield MF, Grunau RV, Linton J and Hadjistavropoulos HD. Pain in the preterm neonate: behavioural and physiological indices (published erratum appears in *Pain* 1993 Jul;**54**(1):111). *Pain* 1993;**52**:287–299.

25. Barrier G, Attia J, Mayer MN, Amiel TC and Shnider SM. Measurement of post-operative pain and narcotic administration in infants using a new clinical scoring system. *Intensive Care Med* 1989;**15**:S37–39.

26. Anand KJ, Hansen DD and Hickey PR. Hormonal–metabolic stress responses in neonates undergoing cardiac surgery. *Anesthesiology* 1990;**73**:661–670.

27. Pokela ML. Effect of opioid-induced analgesia on beta-endorphin, cortisol and glucose responses in neonates with cardiorespiratory problems. *Biol Neonate* 1993;**64**:360–367.

28. Quinn MW, Wild J, Dean HG et al. Randomised double-blind controlled trial of effect of morphine on catecholamine concentrations in ventilated pre-term babies. *Lancet* 1993;**342**:324–327.

29. Anand KJ, Sippell WG and Aynsley GA. Randomised trial of fentanyl anaesthesia in preterm babies undergoing surgery: effects on the stress response. *Lancet* 1987;**1**:62–66.

30. Franck LS and Gregory GA. Clinical evaluation and treatment of infant pain in the neonatal intensive care unit. In: Schechter NL, Berde CB and Yaster M (eds) *Pain in Infants, Children, and Adolescents*. Baltimore: Williams & Wilkins, 1993:519–535.

31. Harpin VA and Rutter N. Making heel pricks less painful. *Arch Dis Child* 1983;**58**:226–228.

32. Blass EM and Hoffmeyer LB. Sucrose as an analgesic for newborn infants. *Pediatrics* 1991;**87**:215–218.

33. Rushforth JA and Levene MI. Effect of sucrose on crying in response to heel stab. *Arch Dis Child* 1993;**69**:388–389.

34. Rushforth JA, Griffith G, Thorpe H and Levene MI. Can topical lignocaine reduce behavioural response to heel prick? *Arch Dis Child* 1995;**72**:F49–51.

35. Wester U. Analgesic effect of lidocaine ointment on intact skin in neonates. *Acta Paediatr* 1993;**82**:791.

36. McIntosh N, van Veen L and Brameyer H. Alleviation of the pain of heel prick in preterm infants. *Arch Dis Child* 1994;**70**:F177–181.

37. Stang HJ, Gunnar MR, Snellman L, Condon LM and Kestenbaum R. Local anesthesia for neonatal circumcision. Effects on distress and cortisol response. *JAMA* 1988;**259**:1507–1511.

38. Howard CR, Howard FM and Weitzman ML. Acetaminophen analgesia in neonatal circumcision: the effect on pain. *Pediatrics* 1994;**93**:641–646.

39. Pokela ML. Pain relief can reduce hypoxemia in distressed neonates during routine treatment procedures. *Pediatrics* 1994;**93**:379–383.

40. Anand KJ and Hickey PR. Halothane–morphine compared with high-dose sufentanil for anesthesia and postoperative analgesia in neonatal cardiac surgery. *N Engl J Med* 1992;**326**:1–9.

41. Porter FL, Miller JP, Cole FS and Marshall RE. A controlled clinical trial of local anesthesia for lumbar punctures in newborns. *Pediatrics* 1991;**88**:663–669.

42. Marchette L, Main R, Redick E, Bagg A and Leatherland J. Pain reduction interventions during neonatal circumcision. *Nurs Res* 1991;**40**:241–244.

43. Weatherstone KB, Rasmussen LB, Erenberg A, Jackson EM, Claflin KS and Leff RD. Safety and efficacy of a topical anesthetic for neonatal circumcision. *Pediatrics* 1993;**92**:710–714.

44. Bucher HU, Moser T, von Siebenthal K, Keel M, Wolf M and Duc G. Sucrose reduces pain reaction to heel lancing in preterm infants. *Pediatr Res* 1995;**38**:332–335.

45. Barrett DA and Rutter N. Percutaneous lignocaine absorption in newborn infants. *Arch Dis Child* 1994;**71**:F122–124.

46. Nilsson A, Engberg G, Henneberg S, Danielson K and De Verdier CH. Inverse relationship between age-dependent erythrocyte activity of methaemoglobin reductase and prilocaine-induced methaemoglobinaemia during infancy. *Br J Anaesth* 1990;**64**:72–76.

47. Yaster M, Tobin JR, Fisher QA and Maxwell LG. Local anesthetics in the management of acute pain in children. *J Pediatr* 1994;**124**:165–176.

48. Welborn LG, Rice LJ, Hannallah RS, Broadman LM, Ruttimann UE and Fink R. Postoperative apnea in former preterm infants: prospective comparison of spinal and general anesthesia. *Anesthesiology* 1990;**72**:838–842.

49. Maunuksela EL. Nonsteroidal anti-inflammatory drugs in pediatric pain management. In: Schechter JL, Berde CB and Yaster M (eds) *Pain in Infants, Children, and Adolescents.* Williams & Wilkins, 1993:135–143.

50. Hopkins CS, Underhill S and Booker PD. Pharmacokinetics of paracetamol after cardiac surgery. *Arch Dis Child* 1990;**65**:971–976.

51. Rumack BH and Peterson RG. Acetaminophen overdose: incidence, diagnosis, and management in 416 patients. *Pediatrics* 1978;**62**(suppl.): 898–903.

52. Stuart MJ, Gross SJ, Elrad H and Graeber JE. Effects of acetylsalicylic-acid ingestion on maternal and neonatal hemostasis. *N Engl J Med* 1982; **307**:909–912.

53. Hurwitz ES, Barrett MJ, Bregman D et al. Public Health Service study of Reye's syndrome and medications. Report of the main study (published erratum appears in *JAMA* 1987 Jun 26;257(24):3366). *JAMA* 1987;**257**:1905–1911.

54. Choonara IA, McKay P, Hain R and Rane A. Morphine metabolism in children. *Br J Clin Pharmacol* 1989;**28**:599–604.
55. Bhat R, Chari G, Gulati A, Aldana O, Velamati R and Bhargava H. Pharmacokinetics of a single dose of morphine in preterm infants during the first week of life. *J Pediatr* 1990;**117**:477–481.
56. Chay PC, Duffy BJ and Walker JS. Pharmacokinetic–pharmacodynamic relationships of morphine in neonates. *Clin Pharmacol Ther* 1992; **51**:334–342.
57. McRorie TI, Lynn AM, Nespeca MK, Opheim KE and Slattery JT. The maturation of morphine clearance and metabolism (published erratum appears in *Am J Dis Child* 1992 Nov;**146**(11):1305). *Am J Dis Child* 1992;**146**:972–976.
58. Pokela ML, Olkkola KT, Koivisto M and Ryhanen P. Pharmacokinetics and pharmacodynamics of intravenous meperidine in neonates and infants. *Clin Pharmacol Ther* 1992;**52**:342–349.
59. Greeley WJ and de Bruin NP. Changes in sufentanil pharmacokinetics within the neonatal period. *Anesth Analg* 1988;**67**:86–90.
60. Gauntlett IS, Fisher DM, Hertzka RE, Kuhls E, Spellman MJ and Rudolph C. Pharmacokinetics of fentanyl in neonatal humans and lambs: effects of age. *Anesthesiology* 1988;**69**:683–687.
61. Koehntop DE, Rodman JH, Brundage DM, Hegland MG and Buckley JJ. Pharmacokinetics of fentanyl in neonates. *Anesth Analg* 1986;**65**:227–232.
62. Marlow N, Weindling AM, Van Peer A and Heykants J. Alfentanil pharmacokinetics in preterm infants. *Arch Dis Child* 1990;**65**:349–351.
63. Hartley R, Green M, Quinn M and Levene MI. Pharmacokinetics of morphine infusion in premature neonates. *Arch Dis Child* 1993;**69**:55–58.
64. Dahlstrom B, Bolme P, Feychting H, Noack G and Paalzow L. Morphine kinetics in children. *Clin Pharmacol Ther* 1979;**26**:354–365.
65. Koren G, Butt W, Pape K and Chinyanga H. Morphine-induced seizures in newborn infants. *Vet Hum Toxicol* 1985;**27**:519–520.
66. Yaster M and Maxwell LG. Opioid agonists and antagonists. In: Schechter NL, Berde CB and Yaster M (eds) *Pain in Infants, Children and Adolescents*. Baltimore: Williams & Wilkins, 1993:145–171.
67. Streisand JB, Stanley TH, Hague B, van Vreeswijk H, Ho GH and Pace NL. Oral transmucosal fentanyl citrate premedication in children. *Anesth Analg* 1989;**69**:28–34.
68. Yaster M and Deshpande JK. Management of pediatric pain with opioid analgesics. *J Pediatr* 1988;**113**:421–429.

7

Antenatal Hormone Treatment to Prevent Lung Disease in the Preterm Infant

Roberta A. Ballard

INTRODUCTION

Liggins[1] was the first to observe accelerated maturation of the fetal lung after administration of glucocorticoids, and also the first[2] to publish a large randomized double blind clinical trial of administration of antenatal corticosteroids (ANCS). The mechanisms of accelerated organ maturation with corticosteroids have been extensively studied in the whole animal as well as at the cellular and molecular level[3]. Since 1972, more than 25 randomized trials of ANCS have been done and selected studies have been subjected to meta-analyses[4]. A cumulative meta-analysis of the studies was presented by Sinclair[5] at the NIH Consensus Conference on *Effect of Corticosteroids for Fetal Maturation on Perinatal Outcomes* which was held in 1994. The recommendations of the panel at that conference are included as Table 7.1[6]. In summary, the panel stated: 'antenatal corticosteroid therapy is indicated for women at risk of premature delivery with few exceptions and will result in a substantial decrease in neonatal morbidity and mortality, as well as substantial savings in health care costs. The use of antenatal corticosteroids for fetal maturation is a rare example of a technology that yields substantial cost savings in addition to improving health.'

Table 7.1 Recommendations of the NIH Consensus Panel for Use of Antenatal Corticosteroids (ANCS)

- All fetuses between 24 and 34 weeks gestation at risk of preterm delivery are candidates
- Decision to treat not altered by fetal race or gender or availability of surfactant
- Benefits to fetuses at risk of preterm delivery vastly outweigh the potential risks
- Benefits include a reduction in the risk of respiratory distress syndrome (RDS), mortality and intraventricular haemorrhage (IVH)
- Patients eligible for therapy with tocolytics are eligible for treatment
- Treatment consists of two doses of 12 mg of betamethasone given intramuscularly 24 hours apart or four doses of 6 mg of dexamethasone given intramuscularly 12 hours apart
- Optimal benefit begins 24 hours after initiation of therapy and lasts at least 7 days
- Treatment for <24 hours is associated with significant reductions in mortality, RDS and IVH
- ANCS should be given unless immediate delivery is anticipated (<6 hours)
- ANCS use is recommended in preterm premature rupture of membranes at <30–32 weeks gestation in the absence of clinical chorioamnionitis
- In complicated pregnancies where delivery before 34 weeks gestation is likely, ANCS use is recommended unless there is evidence that corticosteroids will have an adverse effect on the mother

GLUCOCORTICOID EFFECTS

Although initial studies on the effects of ANCS focused on maturation of the lung[3,7] (Table 7.2) data have accumulated from both animal and human studies that ANCS administration is also the most effective way to prevent intraventricular haemorrhage[4,8–11]. In addition, ANCS administration potentiates the beneficial response to surfactant replacement[12–14] and matures the sympathoadrenal and cardiovascular responses of the preterm animal and human[9,15–18]. There are animal data and some clinical observations suggesting that

Table 7.2 Maturational effects of glucocorticoids on the developing lung

- Increase in both total tissue and alveolar surfactant pools
- Decrease in vascular permeability with less protein leak into the alveolar spaces
- Enhancement of clearance of lung water
- Upregulation of antioxidant enzyme activity
- Maturation of parenchymal structure
- Increase in lung compliance and maximal lung volume
- Enhancement of the response to surfactant treatment
- Improvement in respiratory function and survival

ANCS also reduce the incidence of necrotizing enterocolitis[19,20] and patent ductus arteriosus[9,21–23] in treated infants.

The level of unbound (active) corticosteroid to which the fetus is exposed[24] (Figure 7.1) is virtually the same as the physiological stress response that occurs in the untreated premature infant who develops respiratory distress syndrome (RDS). Thus, antenatal therapy 'starts the clock' for preparing the lung for air breathing. Infants treated in utero with a single course of ANCS do not have evidence of adrenal suppression and have an appropriate response in corticosteroid levels when exposed to stress after birth. Hetherington and Soll did a meta-analysis of the two recommended treatment regimens (see Table 7.1) and found each was associated with a similar statistically significant decrease in RDS, but that the reduction in mortality is significant for betamethasone but not for dexamethasone[7].

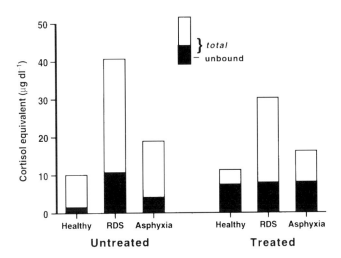

Figure 7.1 The data represent measured values for endogenous cortisol and calculated unbound glucocorticoid activity (cortisol plus betamethasone) in untreated infants and treated infants delivered immediately after a second dose of betamethasone (acetate/phosphate) when betamethasone levels would be highest and cortisol lowest. Untreated infants increase their cortisol in response to intrapartum asphyxia and in response to developing RDS after birth. Despite suppression of their cortisol at birth, treated infants also have a substantial increase in their endogenous cortisol concentrations in response to either asphyxia or RDS. The maximal level of glucocorticoid activity in treated infants (7–8 μg dl⁻¹) is comparable with the physiological stress response level achieved in untreated infants with RDS.

OTHER AGENTS INVESTIGATED FOR PREVENTION OF LUNG DISEASE

A number of other agents have been investigated both in the laboratory and in clinical studies[25] (Table 7.3) Most interest has centred on thyroid hormone and thyrotrophin releasing hormone (TRH)[26]. In 1973, Wu et al[27] found that T4 treated rabbit fetuses had better air retention, more surface-active material in lung fluid, and enhanced morphological development by both light and electron microscopy. In the pregnant rat, T3 therapy stimulates the rate of choline incorporation into phosphatidylcholine by fetal lung and increases the activity of the enzyme cholinephosphate cytidyltransferase in lung tissue[28], without a change in endogenous corticosterone concentration. Studies in culture systems have established that fetal lung is a direct target tissue for thyroid hormones. Tri-iodothyronine (T3) and thyroxine (T4) stimulate the rate of precursor incorporation into phosphatidylcholine and phosphatidylglycerol in organ cultures of fetal rat, rabbit and human lung[3]. Chan et al[29] found an improvement in neonatal pulmonary function in fetal lambs who received intra-amniotic T3 without an increase in tracheal phospholipids. In the human, Mashiach et al[30] administered intra-amniotic T4 to women before preterm delivery and found an association with enhanced lung maturity. Subsequently, Schreyer et al[31] and Romaguera et al[32] both attempted to accelerate fetal lung maturation by injection of T3 into the amniotic fluid. They suggested that one week of therapy caused an acceleration of lecithin to sphingomyelin (L:S) ratio maturation and decreased RDS in fetuses of more than 27 weeks gestation in these pregnancies; however, the studies were not randomized and all of the women treated had complicated pregnancies. The controls were women with uncomplicated pregnancies. To date, there have

Table 7.3 Agents investigated for beneficial effect on lung maturation

- Thyroid hormones
- Thyrotrophin-releasing hormone (thyroxine and prolactin released)
- β-Adrenergic agents
- Prolactin
- Oestradiol
- Epidermal growth factor
- Theophylline
- Interferon
- Ambroxol

been no controlled studies of intra-amniotic administration of T3 and it is highly likely that this approach would result in variable fetal absorption of hormone.

COMBINATION OF GLUCOCORTICOIDS WITH THYROID HORMONES

Superadditive and rapid effects of the combination of T3 and dexamethasone on surfactant metabolism in vitro have been well described[28,33] (Figure 7.2). The effect of combined hormonal therapy on both biochemical and morphological differentiation in human fetal lung in tissue culture has also been demonstrated[34] (Figure 7.3). In fetal lambs, treatment with cortisol plus either T3 and prolactin or by TRH (which stimulates the release of T3 and prolactin) was more effective than cortisol alone in accelerating lung structural development and the production of surfactant[35,36]. Schellenberg et al[37] studied the relationship between elastin and collagen concentration and indices of lung maturity in fetal sheep. They suggested that the

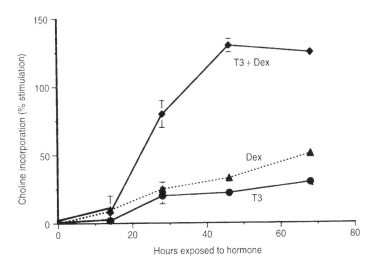

Figure 7.2 Time course of hormonal stimulation. Lungs from 23 day rabbit fetuses were cultured for 68 hours in the absence or presence of hormones. T3 (1 nmol l⁻¹), dexamethasone (Dex) (10 nmol l⁻¹) or T3 plus Dex was added to the cultures for the entire 68 hours or the last 46, 28 or 14 hours of culture. The rate of choline incorporation was determined after 68 hours of culture. Values are means ± SE of triplicate determinations.

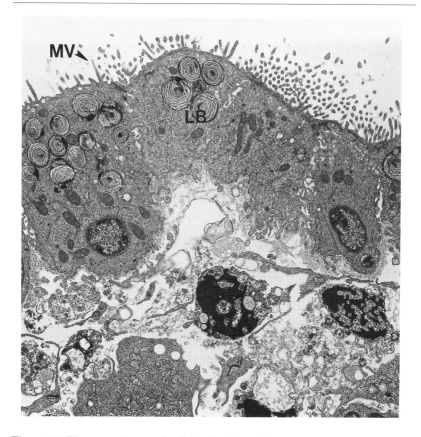

Figure 7.3 Electron micrograph of the alveolar epithelium of an explant from an 18 week gestation lung. After 4 days of culture in the presence of T3 plus dexamethasone, the apical cytoplasm contains many large lamellar bodies (LB), and numerous long microvilli (MV) extend into the alveolar space. Glycogen pools are notably absent (×6900).

increased distensibility of fetal lung in response to antenatal hormones is attributable, in part, to changes in the composition of connective tissue. These observations led clinicians to speculate that combined hormonal therapy might decrease the incidence of chronic lung disease as well as RDS in preterm infants. Warburton et al[38] found additional benefits in the lamb model from the addition of β-agonists to corticosteroid and thyroid hormone. More recently, Ikegami et al[39] observed that treatment with combined corticosteroid and TRH increased the level of surfactant protein-A in alveolar wash fivefold.

Jobe and coworkers are investigating the effects of direct fetal injection of hormones in fetal lambs[40]. Polk et al[41] reported that a single direct fetal exposure to betamethasone 48 hours before delivery results in significant improvement in postnatal pulmonary function. Administration of T4 in combination with corticosteriod results in further augmentation of the effect at 48 but not at 24 hours. The effects occur independent of any effect on surfactant pool sizes and thus probably are indicative of changes in lung structure.

ADMINISTRATION OF COMBINED HORMONAL THERAPY IN THE HUMAN

Maternal administration of either T3 or T4 is not effective as a way to administer thyroid hormone to the fetus because high maternal levels of thyroid binding globulin prevent significant amounts of hormone from crossing the placenta to the fetus. In addition, the placenta expresses *s*-monodeiodinase activity which inactivates maternally derived T4 and T3[42]. TRH, however, is a tripeptide which easily crosses the placenta and stimulates the release of both thyroid hormone and prolactin[43–46].

THYROTROPHIN RELEASING HORMONE

The characteristics of TRH have recently been reviewed by de Zegher et al[47]. TRH was the first discovered hypothalamic releasing hormone, is the smallest peptide hormone and is present in some invertebrate species that lack a pituitary gland. TRH is present as early as 10–12 weeks gestation in the human and the concentration rises toward term. It is found in numerous regions of the nervous system, including the cerebellum, as well as the pancreas, placenta, retina and male reproductive organs. Plasma half life in the non-pregnant adult is very short (7 minutes) but is longer in pregnant women. Administration is associated with the release of thyroxine as well as prolactin, but clearly there is also neurotransmitter release. Side effects of TRH are probably secondary to neurotransmitter effects and include nausea, vomiting, urinary urgency, light headedness, a peculiar taste and, with rapid administration, a transient rise in blood pressure[48–50]. Umans et al[51] found that intravenous administration of TRH in the fetal lamb resulted in behavioural arousal, increased fetal breathing and increased blood pressure. The effects on behaviour, but not breathing, were abolished by mus-carinic blockade.

TRH has been used as a diagnostic agent in both children and adults for more than 20 years[48]. No side effects have been observed in the human fetus, however there is some evidence of a maturational effect on fetal heart rate reactivity and fetal breathing activity[47].

de Zegher et al[52] recently described a mother–infant pair who are both heterozygous for a point mutation affecting the Pit-1 gene, which resulted in growth failure, prolactin deficiency and hypothy-roidism. The term newborn had severe RDS requiring prolonged mechanical ventilation and oxygen therapy consistent with a major effect of TRH deficiency on lung maturation. Ordinarily, maternal thyroid levels would help prevent such severe disease in the new-born[52].

CLINICAL TRIALS OF TRH PLUS ANCS

Morales et al[53] were the first to publish a report of an unblinded trial of administration of TRH plus betamethasone to women in preterm labour at less than 34 weeks gestation. In that study, the reduction in RDS in treated infants from 44 to 28% compared with women receiving betamethasone alone was not statistically significant but the decrease in the number of infants with bronchopulmonary dysplasia from 24 to 8% was ($P<0.05$). Jikihara et al[54] in a study in Osaka, Japan reported less severe RDS in treated very low birthweight infants, and Althabe et al[55] reported a decreased requirement for mechanical ventilation and lower incidence of chronic lung disease in infants with a mean birth weight of less than 1300 g. The complete data for the latter two trials have not been published.

Between 1986 and 1989 a randomized double blind clinical trial of antenatal TRH plus corticosteroid versus corticosteroid alone was conducted in four centres in the United States[49]. In this study 404 women with threatened preterm delivery at less than or equal to 32 weeks gestation received betamethasone plus TRH (four doses of 400 µg at 8 hour intervals) or betamethasone plus placebo (12 mg q. 24 hours × 2). Of the 103 infants who were fully treated (24 hours) and who weighed less than 1500 g, there was a trend towards a decrease in occurrence of severe respiratory distress (12% in TRH and steroid versus 25% in steroid alone; $P=0.11$). Significantly fewer TRH plus steroid treated infants developed chronic lung disease (requirement for supplemental oxygen at 28 days of age) (17.6 versus

43.9% in the control; $P<0.01$) (Figure 7.4). Adverse outcome, defined as death or continuing oxygen requirement, was also significantly less in the combined therapy treated group, both at 28 days

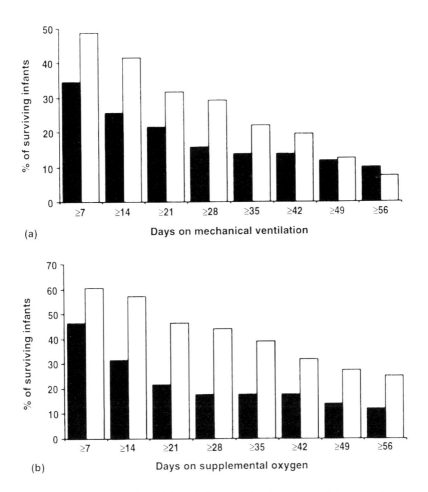

(a)   **Days on mechanical ventilation**

(b)   **Days on supplemental oxygen**

Figure 7.4 Percentage of surviving, fully treated infants in each treatment group requiring assisted ventilation (a) and supplemental oxygen (b) during the first 8 weeks of life. Results are for infants with birthweight ≤1500 g, whose mothers had four doses of TRH or placebo, and who were born less than 10 days after entry into the trial. At 8 weeks, there were 51 survivors of 55 infants in the TRH + steroid (S) group (■) and 40 survivors of 48 infants in the S alone group (□). For days on supplemental oxygen, Wilcox on rank test $P = 0.032$, log rank test $P = 0.042$. (Equivalent statistical tests for days on mechanical ventilation are invalid – see methods.)

Table 7.4 Survival and respiratory status of very low birthweight infants 28 days after birth and at 36 weeks postconception

Liveborn infants	All treated infants		Fully treated infantst	
	TRH + steroid (n = 78)	Steroid-alone (n = 74)	TRH + steroid (n = 55)	Steroid alone (n = 48)
28 days				
Survivors (%)	72 (92.3)	66 (89.2)	51 (92.7)	41 (85.4)
O_2 requirement (%)	16/72 (22.2)	24/66 (36.4)	9/51 (17.6)	18/41 (43.9)*
Adverse outcome (%)‡	22/78 (28.2)	32/74 (43.2)	13/55 (23.6)	25/48 (52.1)*
36 weeks postconception				
Survivors (%)	72 (92.3)	65 (87.8)	51 (92.7)	40 (83.3)
O_2 requirement (%)	10/72 (13.9)	13/65 (20.0)	6/51 (11.8)	10/40 (25.0**)
Adverse outcome (%)‡	16/78 (20.5)	22/74 (29.7)	10/55 (18.2)	18/48 (37.5)*

Values in parentheses are percentages.
† Four doses of TRH or placebo.
‡ Adverse outcome is defined as death or chronic lung disease (requirement for supplemental oxygen).
* $P < 0.01$; ** $P = 0.1$

and when the infants reached 36 weeks post-conceptional age (Table 7.4).

There were, however, several problems with the American study. (1) The design of the study was flawed because the infants of mothers delivering outside the 10 day period following administration of TRH were excluded from analysis, and thus the study did not include 'intention to treat' analysis. Although no deleterious effects on infants born outside the target period were reported, there is no complete knowledge of outcomes for all the infants. (2) None of the infants in the study received surfactant replacement because the study was done during the period of trials of surfactant administration and infants were not enrolled in more than one randomized clinical trial. (3) Although thyroid hormone and TSH levels were obtained on cord blood and in the first few hours of life[46], there was no documentation of later levels or responsiveness of the pituitary thyroid axis. (4) There was a suggestion of an increase in the incidence of patent ductus arteriosus requiring treatment with indomethacin or surgery in infants who received combined hormone treatment. Combination hormone therapy was effective in lowering the incidence of chronic lung disease in both infants with and without patent ductus arteriosus.

Knight et al[56] published the results of a randomized placebo controlled double blind trial (400 μg TRH × 4 and betamethasone 5 mg × 4) in 378 women less than 33 weeks gestation in New Zealand. Of the 405 liveborn infants delivered in the study, 175 were delivered between 24 hours and 10 days of entry. In this subgroup there was a reduction in RDS from 52 to 31% (relative risk 0.61, 95% confidence interval 0.41 to 0.89) and severe respiratory distress from 42 to 20% (RR 0.48, 95% CI 0.29 to 0.78). These investigators also found a decrease in adverse outcome (death or oxygen requirement at 28 days) from 29% in the steroid alone group to 16% with TRH additive therapy (RR 0.55, 95% CI 0.31 to 0.99). Both RDS ($P<0.05$) and severe RDS ($P<0.01$) were decreased in the entire group.

In 1994, Crowther and Alfirevic[57] did a meta-analysis of the status of clinical trials of TRH plus betamethasone (Figure 7.5). Meta-analysis of the data available for the trials demonstrated a decrease in severe RDS and bronchopulmonary dysplasia and a strong trend toward a decrease in RDS after just three doses of TRH (16 hours).

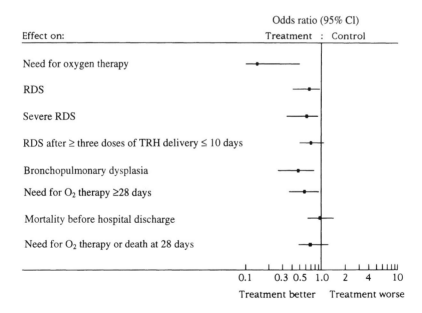

Figure 7.5 Meta-analysis of data from five trials (excluding ACTOBAT), modified from Crowther and Alfirevic[57].

NEURODEVELOPMENTAL OUTCOME

de Zegher at al[58] found evidence of accelerated maturation of somatosensory evoked potentials in preterm infants treated antenatally with TRH/dexamethasone. This acceleration was followed by compensatory relative deceleration in the following week.

Piecuch et al[59] have examined the preschool age neurodevelopmental outcome of a subgroup of the infants in the American study and found no evidence of deleterious effect on either neurological or cognitive outcome.

THE NEED FOR FURTHER STUDIES

A recent larger trial[60] in Australia, the Australian Collaborative Trial of Antenatal Thyrotropin Releasing Hormone (ACTOBAT), entered 1234 women between 24 and 32 weeks gestation into a randomized trial of TRH (200 mg) plus betamethasone versus betamethasone alone. These investigators failed to demonstrate any benefit of combined therapy (Table 7.5) and raised concerns about possible side effects (maternal nausea and vomiting, light headedness and a rise in blood pressure) or risks to the infant (an increase in RDS from 10 to 16% in the infants delivered more than 10 days after therapy). There was no difference in outcome for treated infants versus control infants delivered less than 24 hours after the first dose of drugs.

With regard to the apparent failure to demonstrate efficacy in this trial, it should be noted that, although not statistically significant, there was a trend in the ACTOBAT toward less severe RDS among TRH treated infants delivering <10 days after entry into the trial (24 versus 18%). However, the magnitude of the response is clearly much less than seen in the previous studies and this is indeed puzzling.

One possible explanation is that the investigators used both a lower dose of TRH (200 versus 400 µg) as well as less frequent administration (q. 12 versus 8 hours) compared with other trials. It is possible that their treatment regimen did not sufficiently sustain elevated hormone levels in the fetuses. The increase in fetal TSH and thyroid hormones with TRH administration is transient and levels fall to below control values by 7–12 hours after infusion of TRH. Unfortunately, data are not available for thyroid hormones in cord bloods of infants in the ACTOBAT to address this possibility.

Other possibilities to explain the reduced efficacy in the ACTOBAT might relate to both the antenatal and postnatal use of

Table 7.5 Respiratory and mortality data on outcome of infants who received 'optimal treatment' delivering between 24 hours and 10 days after initiation of therapy and those who delivered more than 10 days after initial therapy

| | 'Optimal treatment' 24 hours–10 days | | | | >10 Days after entry | | | |
	TRH (%) (n=266)	Control (%) (n=240)	RR	95% CI	P	TRH (%) (n=342)	Control (%) (n=366)	RR	95% CI	P
RDS	50	48	1.03	0.86–1.23	0.77	16	10	1.66	1.12–2.46	0.01
Severe RDS	17	22	0.77	0.54–1.07	0.14	6	6	1.07	0.60–1.92	0.82
Need for ventilation	67	62	1.07	0.94–1.22	0.30	17	13	1.34	0.94–1.91	0.10
Oxygen at 28 days	34	34	0.99	0.78–1.26	0.94	8	4	1.74	0.95–3.18	0.07
Death or oxygen at 28 days	41	42	0.98	0.80–1.21	0.88	10	6	1.68	0.99–2.85	0.05
Neonatal death	11	10	1.09	0.65–1.82	0.74	3	1	1.93	0.65–5.69	0.23

Adapted from ACTOBAT[60].

steroids or replacement surfactant. Women in this trial rarely received retreatment (<2%) with antenatal steroids for recurrent premature labour, a practice that was common in other studies. Steroids are also frequently used postnatally to treat established lung disease and this potential confounder was not addressed in their report. Surfactant treatment was introduced in Australia during the period of patient enrolment (after about 25% of the patients had been enrolled). Apparently there were no uniform guidelines for this treatment nor analysis with this important variable as a covariate.

POTENTIAL RISKS OF TRH

The second major conclusion of the ACTOBAT related to perinatal and maternal risk. It should be noted that the two apparent adverse responses of TRH on neonatal outcome (for infants delivering more than 10 days after entry), any RDS and need for ventilation, were both of marginal statistical significance with confidence intervals at 1.0. Most importantly, there was no excess of severe RDS in the TRH group and the duration of ventilation was not different for the two groups. Thus, it is uncertain whether these observations are clinically important.

The maternal findings of nausea and vomiting are known and transient side effects of TRH treatment in adults and have been observed in other prenatal trials. They usually resolve within 15 minutes of administration. Although 49% of treated women in the trial reported nausea, only 8% actually had vomiting. In the control group 13% reported nausea and 3% had vomiting. The increase in blood pressure reported is also of questionable clinical importance. There was an increase in both the number of women with blood pressure $\geq140/90$ mmHg (31 versus 24%; $P = 0.01$) and the number of women with diastolic pressure ≥15 mmHg (23 versus 14%). However, there was no increase in the number of women with blood pressure $\geq160/110$ mmHg. Therefore, although blood pressure increase is potentially of concern, particularly in women with preeclampsia, there have been no reports of clinical problems related to the transient increase. In contrast to the ACTOBAT results, we did not find a significant increase in maternal blood pressure, defined as an increase >20 mmHg[46]. In our study >140/90 was defined as an exclusion criterion, compared with levels of 150/110 in the ACTOBAT.

It is clear that there is a need for additional randomized controlled double blinded studies of this therapeutic intervention which include analysis of the 'intention to treat' group. One such large study, which will enter 1100 women under 30 weeks gestation, is currently underway in 15 sites in North America and another large study is planned to begin in the autumn of 1995 as a pan-European study. These studies will address issues of efficacy in the surfactant treatment era and will carefully look for evidence of deleterious effects in infants delivering less than 24 hours or more than 10 days after therapy. In addition, issues involving the patent ductus arteriosus and responsiveness of the pituitary thyroid axis are being investigated, along with potential mechanisms for the effect on severe RDS and chronic lung disease.

HORMONAL THERAPY FOR CONGENITAL DIAPHRAGMATIC HERNIA

Glick et al[61] and subsequently Wilcox et al[62] described surfactant deficiency in the lamb model of congenital diaphragmatic hernia (CDH) which responded to surfactant therapy. Sullivan et al[63] obtained amniotic fluid for L:S ratios on 18 fetuses with the diagnosis of CDH. They compared the values with published control values for uncomplicated pregnancies and did not find lower L:S ratios or phosphatidylglycerol levels in CDH fetuses. Wilcox et al[64] examined this issue in the lamb model and found that the L:S ratio and phosphatidylglycerol levels in amniotic fluid were not accurate in predicting functional surfactant deficiency after birth. Levels of surfactant proteins have not been examined but may explain this lack of correlation. Further evaluation of this problem in the human is necessary. Suen et al[65] produced a rat model of CDH by administration of nitrofen early in gestation and found that antenatal dexamethasone increased saturated phosphatidylcholine, reduced lung glycogen and produced morphological changes consistent with accelerated maturation. The same investigators[66] described antenatal treatment in this model with combination dexamethasone and TRH. They observed a small but significant improvement in alveolar stability in CDH rats who received combined hormonal therapy over that produced with dexamethasone alone. It is possible that antenatal therapy with steroids and TRH in the human with CDH might be beneficial and probably deserves clinical evaluation.

POTENTIAL MECHANISMS OF ACTION OF COMBINED HORMONAL THERAPY

Several areas of investigation are being pursued in the attempt to understand the mechanism(s) of action of TRH plus glucocorticoids on lung maturation.

The Role for Surfactant Protein-A (SP-A)

Ikegami et al[39] demonstrated a fivefold increase in SP-A in alveolar lavage fluid obtained from fetal lambs at 128 days gestation who were sacrificed 1.25 hours after birth. Yukitake et al[67] recently reported that surfactant protein-A in the rabbit model has a significant protective effect for surfactant against the inhibitory effects of plasma proteins. Carlton et al[68] studied the effect of surfactant administration on fluid balance in the premature lung immediately after birth and found that surfactant administration at birth diminishes transvascular movement of fluid across the pulmonary microcirculation, preserves lung vascular protein permeability and reduces pulmonary oedema. They found a marked increase in protein drainage from both lymph and alveolar space between 2–4 hours before birth and 6–8 hours after birth. One could hypothesize that, although there is maturation of the surfactant system by hormonal therapy, some infants will still have some respiratory distress with leakage of plasma proteins into the alveolar space.

Coalson et al[69] demonstrated a deficiency of SP-A mRNA in their primate model of bronchopulmonary dysplasia and Hallman et al[70] reported that preterm extremely low birthweight ($\leq$1000 g) infants with a low SP-A:saturated phosphatidylcholine ratio during the first postnatal week have higher mortality and morbidity (bronchopulmonary dysplasia) rates. Antenatal stimulation with TRH might result in an increased level of SP-A which would protect surfactant function (either endogenous or administered) in the lungs of these infants, thus resulting in decreased severity of RDS and contributing to decreased chronic lung disease as well. In addition, SP-A appears to play an important role in host defence in the lung[71].

Clearance of Lung Water

Barker et al[72] demonstrated that hormone therapy with dexamethasone and T3 accelerates the normal maturation of the response to catecholamines (resorption of lung fluid) in the fetal lamb lung. In the untreated fetal lamb there is no effect of catecholamines on secretion or reabsorption of lung water until after 130 days gestation. With combined hormonal therapy, however, catecholamines induce resorption of lung liquid as early as 115–118 days. In addition, combined hormonal therapy[73] increases the synthesis of atrial natriuretic factor by alveolar type II cells, which might also contribute to clearance to lung water.

Lung Structural Effects

There is evidence that combined therapy with TRH and corticosteroid results in both improved stability and distensibility of the fetal lung[35,36,38]. Schellenberg et al[37] speculated that the increased distensibility of the fetal lung in response to antenatal combined hormone treatment is due in part to induced changes in the elastin and collagen concentrations in the lung, which mirror the changes that occur during normal development.

Warburton et al[38] found that combined hormone therapy with corticosteroid, TRH and β-agonist produced a 20-fold increase in saturated phosphatidylcholine content of fetal lung lavage and in addition, a threefold increase in lung stability to inflation (measured at V_{40}) and eightfold increase in lung stability to deflation (V_{10}). None of the hormones singly or in double combinations were as effective as triple therapy.

deMello et al[74] have described delayed pulmonary maturation in the hypothyroid (hyt/hyt) mouse. In addition to delay in biochemical maturation, the newborn hyt/hyt lungs had delayed morphological maturation, suggesting that thyroid hormones may play a role in normal lung cytodifferentiation.

Antioxidant Effects

Frank et al[75] demonstrated stimulation of antioxidant enzyme activity by dexamethasone. Chen et al[76] further demonstrated that premature rats treated with TRH plus glucocorticoids tolerated exposure to 95% oxygen with increased antioxidant enzyme levels in the treated group. Thus, although their previous observations had suggested that antioxidant gene expression was lowered by combined hormonal therapy when compared with glucocorticoids alone, it is clear that in the presence of hyperoxia, gene expression is upregulated and there is an increase in protective enzyme levels. The treated group of animals also had less lung oedema after 14 days of hyperoxic exposure compared with the control group.

It is also possible that combined hormonal therapy might have a positive effect on vitamin A metabolism. Vitamin A is known to have a protective effect on development of chronic lung disease in animal models and there is a significant suggestive beneficial effect in the human as well[77].

Effects on Growth or Healing

A number of inflammatory cytokines have been reported to be elevated in chronic lung disease and it is possible that combined hormonal therapy has some effect on inflammatory mediators, either directly or through its effect on SP-A. In addition, one might propose that hormones have an effect on growth factors, such as insulin-like growth factor, or their binding proteins.

Neurotransmitter Effect

As mentioned above and by de Zegher et al[47] in their review, it is well known that TRH also acts as a neurotransmitter in addition to its known endocrine effects. TRH receptors are present in the nucleus tractus solitarius[78] and, therefore, TRH could be involved in control of breathing, and receptors are also present in the limbic system[79], the centre for arousal. Thus, TRH might result in some improved pulmonary mechanics in utero that conceivably could result in improved outcome. In addition, Devaskar et al[80] have suggested that the functional and morphological maturation in the fetal rabbit lung in response to TRH might be, in part or total, mediated through neurotransmitter effects.

SUMMARY

Antenatal therapy with glucocorticoids is a well established, cost effective therapy for reducing morbidity and mortality in the preterm infant. Early studies of the possibility of combined hormonal therapy with TRH and ANCS are promising and results of large multicentre trials currently being conducted in North America and Europe should clarify the risks and benefits of this therapy in the near future.

REFERENCES

1. Liggins GC. Premature delivery of foetal lambs infused with glucocorticoids. *J Endocrinol* 1969;**45**:515–523.
2. Liggins GC and Howie RN. A controlled trial of antepartum glucocorticoid treatment for prevention of the respiratory distress syndrome in premature infants. *Pediatrics* 1972;**50**:515–520.
3. Ballard PL. Hormones and lung maturation. *Monograph on Endocrinology*, vol. 28. Heidelberg: Springer Verlag, 1986; pp 27–198.
4. Crowley P. Update of the antenatal steroid meta-analysis: current knowledge and future research needs. *Am J Obstet Gynecol* 1995;**173**:322–335.
5. Sinclair JC. *Report of the Consensus Development Conference on the Effect of Corticosteroids for Fetal Maturation on Perinatal Outcomes*. NIH Publication 95–3784, November 1994, p. 95.
6. NIH Consensus Development Panel. Consensus Development Conference on the Effect of Corticosteroids for Fetal Maturation on Perinatal Outcomes. *JAMA* 1995;**273**:413–418.
7. Ballard PL and Ballard RA. Scientific basis and therapeutic regimens for use of antenatal glucocorticoids. *Am J Obstet Gynecol* 1995;**173**:254–262.
8. Garite TJ, Rumney PJ, Briggs GG et al. A randomized, placebo-controlled trial of betamethasone for the prevention of respiratory distress syndrome at 24 to 28 weeks gestation. *Am J Obstet Gynecol* 1992;**166**:646–651.
9. Kari MA, Hallman M, Eronen M et al. Prenatal dexamethasone treatment in conjunction with human surfactant therapy. A randomized placebo-controlled multicenter study. *Pediatrics* 1994;**93**:730–736.
10. Shankaran S, Bauer CR, Bain R et al. Relationship between antenatal steroid administration in Grade III and IV intracranial hemorrhage in low birth weight infants. *Am J Obstet Gynecol* 1995;**173**:305–312.
11. Ment LR, Oh W, Ehrenkranz RA, Philip AGS, Duncan CC and Makuch RW. Antenatal steroids, delivery mode, and intraventricular hemorrhage in preterm infants. *Am J Obstet Gynecol* 1995;**172**:795–800.
12. Seidner S, Pettenazzo A, Ikegami M and Jobe A. Corticosteroid potentiation of surfactant dose response in preterm rabbits. *J Appl Physiol* 1988;**64**:2366–2371.
13. Andrews EB, White AD, Weinberg JM, Layne R and Long WA. Antenatal steroids and neonatal outcomes in infants receiving surfactant in the Exosurf treatment IND. *Pediatr Res* 1992;**31**:241 (abstract).
14. Jobe AH, Mitchell BR and Gunkel JH. Beneficial effects of the combined use of prenatal corticosteroids and postnatal surfactant on preterm infants. *Am J Obstet Gynecol* 1993;**168**:508–513.
15. Stein HM, Oyama K, Martinez A et al. Effects of corticosteroids in preterm sheep on adaptation and sympathoadrenal mechanisms at birth. *Am J Physiol* 1993;**264**:E763–769.
16. Collaborative Group on Antenatal Steroid Therapy. Effect of antenatal dexamethasone administration on the prevention of respiratory distress syndrome. *Am J Obstet Gynecol* 1981;**141**:276–286.

17. Leviton A, Kuban KC, Pagano M, Allred EN and Van Marter L. Antenatal corticosteroids appear to reduce the risk of postnatal germinal matrix hemorrhage in intubated low birth weight newborns. *Pediatrics* 1993;**91**:1083–1088.

18. Moise AA, Wearden ME, Welty SE, Kozinetz CA and Hansen TN. Antenatal steroids reduce the need for blood pressure support in extremely premature infants. *Pediatrics* 1995;**95**:845–850.

19. Bauer CR, Morrison JC, Poole WK et al. Decreased incidence of necrotizing enterocolitis after prenatal glucocorticoid therapy. *Pediatrics* 1984;**73**:682.

20. Halac E, Halac J, Beque EF et al. Prenatal and postnatal corticosteroid therapy to prevent neonatal necrotizing enterocolitis: a controlled trial. *J Pediatr* 1990;**117**:132–138.

21. Clyman RI, Ballard PL, Sniderman S et al. Prenatal administration of betamethasone for prevention of patent ductus arteriosus. *J Pediatr* 1981;**98**:123–126.

22. Waffarn F, Siassi B, Cabal LA and Schmidt PL. Effect of antenatal glucocorticoids on clinical closure of the ductus arteriosus. *Am J Dis Child* 1983;**137**:336.

23. Papageorgiou AN, Doray JL and Ardilia R. Reduction of mortality, morbidity and respiratory distress syndrome in infants weighing less than 1000 grams by treatment with betamethasone and ritodrine. *Pediatrics* 1989;**83**:493–497.

24. Ballard PL, Granberg JP and Ballard RA. Glucocorticoid levels in maternal and cord serum after prenatal betamethasone therapy to prevent respiratory distress syndrome. *J Clin Invest* 1975;**56**:1548–1554.

25. Ballard RA and Ballard PL. Lung maturation in prenatal preparation of the fetus. In: Reed GB, Claireaux AE and Cockburn F (eds) *Diseases of the Fetus and Newborn*, 2nd edn. London: Chapman and Hall, 1995:1337–1343.

26. Ballard PL. Hormonal regulation of pulmonary surfactant. *Endocr Rev* 1989;**10**:165–181.

27. Wu B, Kikkawa Y, Roazalesi MM et al. The effect of thyroxine on the maturation of fetal rabbit lungs. *Biol Neonate* 1973;**22**:161–168.

28. Gross I, Dynia DW, Wilson CM et al. Glucocorticoid–thyroid interactions in fetal rat lung. *Pediatr Res* 1984;**18**:191–196.

29. Chan L, Miller T, Winkel C et al. Intra-amniotic tri-iodothyronine (T3) improves neonatal pulmonary function in the preterm lambs. *Soc Gynecol Invest* 1994;(abstract 55).

30. Mashiach S, Barkai G, Sack J et al. The effect of intraamniotic thyroxine administration on fetal lung maturity in man. *J Perinatol Med* 1979;**7**:161–169.

31. Schreyer P, Caspi E, Letko Y, Ron-El R, Pinto N and Zeidman JL. Intraamniotic triiodothyronine instillation for prevention of respiratory distress syndrome in pregnancies complicated by hypertension. *J Perinat Med* 1982;**10**:27.

32. Romageura J, Zorrilla C, de la Vega A et al. Responsiveness of L-S ratio of the amniotic fluid to intra-amniotic administration of thyroxine. *Acta Obstet Gynecol Scand* 1990;**69**:119–122.

33. Ballard PL, Hovey ML and Gonzales LK. Thyroid hormone stimulation of phosphatidylcholine synthesis in cultured fetal rabbit lung. *J Clin Invest* 1984;**74**:898–905.
34. Gonzales LW, Ballard PL, Ertsey R and Williams MC. Glucocorticoids and thyroid hormones stimulate biochemical and morphological differentiation of human fetal lung in organ culture. *J Clin Endocrinol Metab* 1986; **62**:687–691.
35. Liggins GC, Schellenberg JC, Manzai M, Kitterman JA and Lee CCH. Synergism of cortisol and thyrotropin releasing hormone on lung maturation in fetal sheep. *J Appl Physiol* 1988;**65**:1880–1884.
36. Boshier CP, Holloway H, Liggins GC and Marshall RJ. Morphometric analyses of the effects of thyrotropin releasing hormone and cortisol on the lungs of fetal sheep. *J Develop Physiol* 1989;**12**:49–54.
37. Schellenberg JC, Liggins GC, Kittermna JA and Lee CH. Elastin and collagen in the fetal sheep lung. II. Relationship to mechanical properties of the lung. *Pediatr Res* 1987;**22**:339–343.
38. Warburton D, Parton L, Buckley S, Cosico L, Enns G and Saluna T. Combined effects of corticosteroid, thyroid hormones, and β-agonist on surfactant, pulmonary mechanics and β-receptor binding in fetal lamb lung. *Pediatr Res* 1988;**24**:166–170.
39. Ikegami M, Polk D, Tabor B et al. Corticosteroid and thyrotropin-releasing hormone effects on preterm sheep lung function. *J Appl Physiol* 1991;**70**:2268–2278.
40. Jobe AH, Polk D, Ikegami M et al. Lung responses to ultrasound-guided fetal treatments with corticosteroids in preterm lambs. *J Appl Physiol* 1993;**75**:2099–2105.
41. Polk DH, Ikegami M, Jobe AH et al. Postnatal lung function in preterm lambs: effects of a single exposure to betamethasone and thyroid hormones. *Am J Obstet Gynecol* 1995;**172**:872–881.
42. Wu SY, Fisher DA and Polk DH. Maturation of thyroid hormone metabolism. In: Wu SY (ed) *Thyroid Hormone Metabolism: Regulation and Clinical Implications*. Boston: Blackwell Scientific, 1991:293–320.
43. Roti E, Gnudi A, Braverman LE et al. Human cord blood concentrations of thyrotropin-releasing hormone. *J Clin Endocrinol Metab* 1976;**53**:813–817.
44. Moya F, Mena P, Heusser F et al. Response of the maternal, fetal, and neonatal pituitary–thyroid axis to thyrotropin-releasing hormone. *Pediatr Res* 1986;**20**:982–986.
45. Moya F, Mena P, Foradori A, Becerra M, Inzunza A and Germain A. Effect of maternal administration of thyrotropin releasing hormone on the preterm fetal pituitary–thyroid axis. *J Pediatr* 1991;**119**:966–971.
46. Ballard PL, Ballard RA, Creasy RK et al. Respiratory disease in very-low-birthweight infants after prenatal thyrotropin-releasing hormone and glucocorticoid. *Pediatr Res* 1992;**32**:673–678.
47. de Zegher F, Spitz B and Devlieger H. Prenatal treatment with thyrotropin releasing hormone to prevent neonatal respiratory distress. *Arch Dis Child* 1992;**67**:450–454.

48. Jackson IM. Thyrotropin-releasing hormone. *N Engl J Med* 1982; **306:**145–150.

49. Ballard RA, Ballard PL, Creasy RK et al. Respiratory disease in very-low-birthweight infants after prenatal thyrotropin-releasing hormone and glucocorticoid. *Lancet* 1992;**339:**510–515.

50. Peek MJ, Bajoria R, Shennan AH, Dalzell F, deSwiet M and Fisk NM. Hypertensive effect of antenatal thyrotropin-releasing hormone in pre-eclampsia. *Lancet* 1995;**345:**793.

51. Umans JG, Umans HR and Szeto HH. Effects of thyrotropin-releasing hormone in the fetal lamb. *Am J Obstet Gynecol* 1986;**155:**1266–1271.

52. de Zegher F, Pernasetti F, Vanhole C, Devlieger H and Martial JA. Fetal immaturity and maternal alactogenesis in fetomaternal Pit-1 deficiency. *J Clin Endocrinol Metab* 1995;**80:**3127–3130.

53. Morales WJ, O'Brien WJ, Angel JF, Knuppel A and Sawai S. Fetal lung maturation: the combined use of corticosteroids and thyrotropin-releasing hormone. *Obstet Gynecol* 1989;**73:**116.

54. Jikihara H, Sawada Y, Imai S et al. Maternal administration of thyro-tropin-releasing hormone for prevention of neonatal respiratory distress syndrome. *6th Congress of the Federation of Asia-Oceana Perinatal Societies*, Perth, Australia 1990; abstract 87.

55. Althabe F, Fustinana C, Althabe O and Cernadas JMC. Controlled trial of prenatal betamethasone plus TRH vs. betamethasone plus placebo for pre-vention of RDS in preterm infants. *Pediatr Res* 1991;**29:**200 (abstract).

56. Knight DB, Liggins GC and Wealthall SR. A randomized controlled trial of antepartum thyrotropin-releasing hormone and betamethasone in the pre-vention of respiratory disease in preterm infants. *Am J Obstet Gynecol* 1994;**171:**11–16.

57. Crowther CA and Alfirevic Z. Antenatal thyrotropin-releasing hormone (TRH) prior to preterm delivery. In: Enkin MW, Keirse MJNC, Renfrew MJ and Neilson JP (eds) *Pregnancy and Childbirth Module*, Cochrane Database of Systematic Reviews: Review No. 2955, 26 April 1993. Published through Cochrane Updates on Disk, Oxford. Update Software, Spring 1993.

58. de Zegher F, deVries L, Pierrat V, Caniels H and Spitz B. Effect of prenatal bethamethasone/thyrotropin releasing hormone treatment on somatosen-sory evoked potentials in preterm newborns. *Pediatr Res* 1992;**32:**212–214.

59. Piecuch R, Ballard R, Leonard C, Behle M and Henning D. Neurodevelopmental outcome of preterm infants treated with antenatal thyrotropin releasing hormone (TRH). *Pediatr Res* 1994;**35:**283 (abstract).

60. Crowther CA, Hiller JE, Haslam RR, Robinson JS and Group AS. Australian collaborative trial of antenatal thyrotropin-releasing hormone (ACTOBAT) for prevention of neonatal respiratory disease. *Lancet* 1995;**345:**877–882.

61. Glick PL, Stannard VA, Leach CL et al. Pathophysiology of congenital diaphragmatic hernia. II. The fetal lamb model is surfactant deficient. *J Pediatr Surg* 1992;**27:**382–388.

62. Wilcox DT, Glick PL, Karamanoukian H, Rossman J, Morin FC and Holm BA. Pathophysiology of congenital diaphragmatic hernia. V. Effect of exogenous surfactant therapy on gas exchange and lung mechanics in the lamb congenital diaphragmatic hernia model. *J Pediatr* 1994; **124:**289–293.

63. Sullivan KM, Hawgood S, Flake AW, Harrison MR and Adzick NS. Amniotic fluid phospholipid analysis in the fetus with congenital diaphragmatic hernia. *J Pediatr Surg* 1994;**29:**1020–1024.

64. Wilcox DT, Glick PL, Karamanoukian HL, Azizkhan RG and Holm BA. Pathophysiology of congenital diaphragmatic hernia XII: Amniotic fluid lecithin/sphingomyelin ratio and phosphatidylglycerol concentrations do not predict surfactant status in congenital diaphragmatic hernia. *J Pediatr Surg* 1995;**30:**410–412.

65. Suen HC, Bloch KD and Donahoe PK. Antenatal glucocorticoid corrects pulmonary immaturity in experimentally induced congenital diaphragmatic hernia in rats. *Pediatr Res* 1994;**35:**523–529.

66. Losty PD, Suen HC, Manganaro TF, Donahoe PK and Schnitzer JJ. Prenatal hormonal therapy improves pulmonary compliance in the nitrifen-induced CDH rat model. *J Pediatr Surg* 1995;**30:**420–426.

67. Yukitake K, Brown CL, Schulueter MA, Clements JA and Hawgood S. Surfactant apoprotein A modifies the inhibitory effect of plasma proteins on surfactant activity in vivo. *Pediatr Res* 1995;**37:**21–25.

68. Carlton DP, Cho SC, Davis P, Lont M and Bland RD. Surfactant treatment at birth reduces lung vascular injury and edema in preterm lambs. *Pediatr Res* 1995;**37:**265–270.

69. Coalson JJ, King RJ, Yang F et al. SP-A deficiency in primate model of bronchopulmonary dysplasia with infection. In situ mRNA and immuno-stains. *Am J Respir Crit Care Med* 1995;**151:**584–566.

70. Hallman M, Merritt A, Akino T and Bry K. Surfactant protein A, phosphatidylcholine, and surfactant inhibitors in epithelial lining fluid. *Am Rev Respir Dis* 1991;**144:**1376–1384.

71. Kuroki Y and Voelker DR. Pulmonary surfactant proteins. Minireview. *J Biol Chem* 1994;**269:**25943–25946.

72. Barker PM, Markiewicz M, Parker KA, Walters DV and Strang LB. Synergistic action of triiodothyronine and hydrocortisone on epinephrine-induced reabsorption of fetal lung liquid. *Pediatr Res* 1990; **27:**588–591.

73. Matsubara M, Mori Y, Umeda Y, Oikawa S, Nakazato H and Inada M. Atrial natriuretic peptide gene expression and its secretion. *Biochem Biophys Res Commun* 1988;**156:**619–627.

74. deMello DE, Heyman S, Govindarajan R, Sosenko IRS and Devaskar UP. Delayed ultrastructural lung maturation in the fetal and newborn hypothyroid (hyt/hyt) mouse. *Pediatr Res* 1994;**36:**380–386.

75. Frank L, Lewis PL and Sosenko IRS. Dexamethasone stimulation of fetal rat lung antioxidant enzyme activity in parallel with surfactant stimulation. *Pediatrics* 1985;**75:**569–574.

76. Chen Y, Sosenko I and Frank L. Positive regulation of antioxidant enzyme gene expression by prenatal TRH plus dexamethasone treatment in premature rat lung exposed to prolonged hyperoxia. *Pediatr Res* 1994;**37**:611–616.

77. Shenai JP, Kennedy KA, Chytil F and Stahlman MT. Clinical trial of vitamin A supplementation in infants susceptible to bronchopulmonary dysplasia. *J Pediatr* 1987;**111**:269–277.

78. Dekin MS, Richerson GB and Getting PA. Thyrotropin-releasing hormone induces rhythmic bursting in neurons of the nucleus tractus solitarius. *Science* 1985;**229**:67–69.

79. Bennet L, Gluckman PD and Johnston BM. The central effects of thyrotropin-releasing hormone on the breathing movements and electrocortical activity of the fetal sheep. *Pediatr Res* 1988;**23**:72–75.

80. Devaskar U, deMello D and Ackerman J. Effect of maternal administration of TRH or DN1417 on functional and morphologic fetal rabbit lung maturation and duration of survival after premature delivery. *Biol Neonate* 1991;**59**:346–351.

8

Systematic Reviews of Randomized Trials in Neonatology

John C. Sinclair

INTRODUCTION

The practice of evidence based neonatology requires efficient access to up to date, valid evidence concerning the efficacy and safety of treatments. One method of keeping abreast of evidence is to consult review articles. Unfortunately, the scientific quality of review articles is often poor, in that they do not regularly use scientific methods to identify, evaluate and synthesize information[1,2]. As a result, it is not surprising that different reviewers sometimes come to different conclusions and make different inferences when reviewing the same topic. Moreover, reviewers may lack efficient methods of detecting shifts in the weight of evidence, leading to a long gap between the time when treatment efficacy has in fact been established and the time when the treatment is routinely recommended in review articles or textbooks[3].

During the past ten years, an increased awareness has developed of the need for scientifically valid reviews in all fields of medical endeavour. In the field of therapy it is now well appreciated that effects of only moderate size nevertheless can be clinically very important. To have sufficient power to detect such treatment effects, a review of *all* relevant and valid studies is required. Moreover, avoidance of bias is essential, particularly in detecting differences of moderate size, so reviews of therapy need primarily to review evidence from randomized trials[4].

In this chapter the methodology of a systematic review incorporating meta-analysis will be briefly presented. The term 'systematic review' is used to distinguish it from a non-systematic review that mixes together opinion and evidence. The term 'meta-analysis' is used to describe the explicit, quantitative steps of summarizing the results of a set of individual trials. The application in the field of neonatology/perinatology of systematic reviews with meta-analysis will be demonstrated.

METHODOLOGY OF SYSTEMATIC REVIEWS

The Research Question

Undertaking a systematic review is a scientific activity. Systematic reviews can be viewed as retrospective research; they are thus subject to many of the same biases which may affect other retrospective studies. Therefore, a high degree of scientific rigour is required of the review process. As for any scientific activity, the methods must be specified in advance and described in the report of the research. The steps in developing a protocol are given in Table 8.1.

The first step in a systematic review is to state, a priori, the research question(s). For reviews of a therapy, just as for the primary studies of a therapy, the research question typically will specify the population, the intervention and the outcomes. A research question that is explicit and focused will inform each stage of the review; it will determine where to look for relevant studies, what primary studies are relevant, what data within each study are relevant, what aspects of methodological quality are critical, and what form of analysis is appropriate.

Table 8.1 Systematic reviews of therapy: developing the protocol

1. Pose the research question explicitly, specifying the population, intervention and outcomes (both beneficial and harmful) of interest
2. Specify the methods used to search for all potentially relevant studies, to select relevant data, to assess its methodologic quality, and to analyse it
3. Specify hypothesis-testing primary and secondary analyses a priori

Adapted from Cook et al[5].

The reviewer frequently will set secondary objectives in addition to the primary research question – for example, subgroup analyses or analyses of sources of variation in the results of the primary studies. Sources of variation might include differences in the populations, in the way the intervention was given, in the definition or method of ascertainment of outcomes, or in other aspects of research design. The scientific value of the review is strengthened when such secondary analyses are specified a priori.

Of course, there is an opportunity in the review process, as in analysing primary studies, for analyses to be undertaken that are suggested by the data rather than determined by the a priori research question and the resulting research protocol. The distinction between such data driven analyses, directed to hypothesis generation, and protocol driven analyses, directed to hypothesis testing, must be made clear in the report of the review.

Identifying and Selecting Studies

Table 8.2 lists the important steps in identifying and selecting the primary reports of research that are relevant to the review.

Table 8.2 Identification and selection of relevant studies

---

1. Consider all relevant sources:
     computerized bibliographic databases: MEDLINE, other
     review articles
     registers
     abstracts
     conference/symposia proceedings
     granting agencies
     industry
     books, dissertations
2. Specify inclusion criteria:
     base selection on a priori specification of population, intervention, outcomes and study design
3. Specify any constraints in study selection:
     inclusion or exclusion of completed but unpublished studies
     language of publication
4. Assess reproducibility of inclusion/exclusion decisions
5. Report methods and results of study selection:
     search strategies used
     studies included, excluded
     agreement

Adapted from Cook and Sackett[5].

Sources of evidence

The objective in identifying relevant evidence for a systematic review is to conduct a search that is comprehensive, i.e. that maximizes sensitivity. In most fields of medicine, including neonatology, the relevant evidence is voluminous and is contained in many different places. For example, there are presently over 3000 reports of randomized trials in neonatology (a number which is doubling every 6 years) and these reports are distributed across many different medical journals. It is clearly impossible to identify these reports by relying on manual searching methods. Thus, electronic searching of computerized bibliographic databases has emerged as probably the most powerful strategy for detecting relevant evidence.

The most important database for reports of biomedical research in most fields, including neonatology, is MEDLINE. MEDLINE contains over six million references to reports from over 4000 biomedical journals dating from 1966 to the present. MEDLINE can be searched economically and efficiently using a software program such as GRATEFUL MED. Using appropriate medical subject headings (MeSH terms) and textwords, the user can carry out a comprehensive search for reports on the biomedical topic of interest. Using methodological 'hedges', the user then can prune the list of on-topic reports to only those that meet specified methodological criteria. For example, if the user wishes to restrict the retrieval to randomized trials, he or she can incorporate into the search strategy MeSH terms or textwords which are sensitive detectors of randomized trials[6].

Table 8.3 lists the methodological terms that have been found to be the most sensitive for detecting randomized trials in the 1990s[7]. The performance of various methodological terms was tested by comparing the yield of electronic searches incorporating such terms with hand search retrieval. Electronic searching of the current literature

Table 8.3 Electronic search-term combination with best sensitivity for detecting randomized controlled trials (1991 onwards)

Randomized controlled trial (pt)
or Drug therapy (sh)
or Therapeutic use (sh)
or Random (tw)

pt, publication type; sh, subheading; tw, textword.
From Haynes et al[7].

indexed in MEDLINE can detect up to 99% of randomized trials of treatment of adult diseases reported in core journals[7]. Sensitivity in detecting trials in neonatology may well be lower because such trials may not be indexed as accurately or completely; further study of this is required. Thus, exclusive reliance on electronic searching cannot yet be recommended.

Publication bias

Having identified all (or virtually all) published reports of research relevant to the question, the reviewer needs also to consider whether to include reports of completed but unpublished research. This question arises not only out of a desire to increase power but, more cogently, because of possible publication bias.

Publication bias arises when the results of the study influence the likelihood of an investigator submitting or a journal accepting a study for publication. There is some evidence that studies with statistically significant results may be more likely to see the light of day than those with 'no difference' results[8–10]. To the extent that it is present, such publication bias can lead to systematic error in reviews of research that rely only on published studies.

Whether or not to include unpublished data in systematic reviews is a controversial issue at present[11]. An obvious difficulty is identifying all unpublished studies, or at least a representative sample. Prospective registries of clinical trials may provide a solution to this problem in future[12,13]. If unpublished studies are included in a systematic review, they must be subjected, of course, to the same rigorous methodological review (see below) as published studies.

Reproducibility of assessments

It is evident that at each stage of the conduct of a systematic review there is an opportunity for non-agreement, either within-rater or among different individuals attempting the same task. Thus, for example, different individuals may not retrieve the same articles on a literature search, or retain the same articles after having applied inclusion/exclusion criteria. Other opportunities for non-agreement arise in later stages (see below), including the steps of validity assessments and data extraction.

Such non-agreement at each step of a systematic review can be described and measured; its sources can be identified and steps taken to minimize it (e.g. blinding to the identity of authors, institution, journal of publication; resolution of discrepancies through discussion and consensus).

Description of methods

A systematic review is a scientific activity having explicit methodology; thus, the report of the review should contain a 'Methods' section. Here the reviewer describes the methods used at each step of the review process, including those concerned with each aspect of study identification and selection that has been discussed. Studies excluded, and the reasons for their exclusion, should be stated. Each element of the methodology used in later steps of the systematic review should similarly be stated.

Assessment of Validity of Primary Studies

A systematic review of a therapy seeks evidence preferably from randomized clinical trials. The randomized trial, compared with research designs using either historical or non-randomized concurrent controls, offers maximum protection against selection bias at entry[14–16]. However, the performance of a randomized trial is not a sufficient guarantee of a valid result. Bias can intrude at multiple points in a trial: at entry, in administering the experimental or control treatment, in determining the outcome and in analysing the data. Therefore, the validity of each primary trial needs to be considered and assessed (Table 8.4).

Objective assessment of the methodological quality of the primary studies requires that a systematic scheme be applied for assessing validity. Methodological standards for the design, conduct, analyses and reporting of randomized trials provide a basis for rating of valid-

Table 8.4 Methodological quality assessment of primary studies

---

1. Base quality assessments on the extent to which bias is minimized:
    method of allocation
    blinding of intervention
    completeness of follow up
    blinding of outcome measurements
2. Distinguish methodological quality of the study from quality of reporting
3. Evaluate the reproducibility of methodological quality assessments
4. Report the methodological scoring system utilized
5. Consider use of methodological quality assessment:
    as a threshold for inclusion in the systematic review
    as a contributor to heterogeneity
    in sensitivity analyses

Adapted from Cook et al[5].

ity[17,18]. However, there is not general agreement on the weights to be put on different elements. There is evidence that control of selection bias at entry is a critical requirement for validity[15]. This is accomplished by blinding the randomization process so that neither clinician nor patient can predict which treatment will be allocated. Blinding of randomization is particularly important when there are good prognostic indices at entry which predict the patient's risk for the target outcome. However, other elements of trial design (such as complete follow up, blinding of the outcome measurement and, where possible, of the intervention) are also critically important, and their relative importance can vary with the nature of the clinical problem. For example, blinding of the intervention is especially important in order to avoid co-intervention bias in clinical situations where effective co-interventions (additional screening, diagnostic or therapeutic interventions) are available. Completeness of follow up is especially important when the target outcome is uncommon or rare. Blinding of the measurement of outcome is especially important for 'soft' outcomes whose measurement is subject to observer variation.

Until there is actual validation of the relative weights to be attached to the different contributors to the validity of trial design, it may be best simply to describe the methodological features of each trial and include these evaluations in the review. (See, for example, the tables to be found as an appendix to each chapter in *Effective Care of the Newborn Infant*[19], in which the reviewer reports critical methodological features of each trial cited in each review.)

Deficiencies in the reports of clinical trials have been documented repeatedly[20-22]. Deficiencies in reporting should be distinguished from defects in trial design and/or conduct. For example, if the method of randomization is not described, or if the presence or absence of blinding is not stated in situations where it is feasible to blind, an assessment of 'can't tell' is appropriate (see, for example, reference 19). Current proposals for improving the quality of trial reporting[23,24] may do much to improve reporting deficiencies in future.

If the methodological quality of trials is summarized qualitatively or quantitatively using an overall score for each trial, a threshold score can be used as an inclusion/exclusion criterion for the systematic review. Additionally, the score can be used as a basis for exploring trial quality as a potential contributor to heterogeneity of results among the set of trials contributing to the review, or as a basis for exploring the sensitivity of the overall result of the review to inclusion/exclusion of trials of varying quality[25].

Combining Results of Independent Studies

Data extraction
The next step in a systematic review is the extraction of data from each study. Outcome data should include data on each of the outcomes, beneficial or harmful, specified by the research question. It is sometimes necessary to contact the original investigators in order to clarify uncertainties (e.g. in patient characteristics, details of interventions, definitions of outcomes) or obtain data that were obtained but are missing from the published report (e.g. outcomes ascertained but not reported, individual patient data needed for analysis by subgroups). Care should be taken to ensure that the process of data extraction is shielded from bias and is reproducible.

Data analysis

Choice of treatment effect estimator (Table 8.5).   The results of randomized trials are important not only as hypothesis tests but also as the preferred source of valid data for forming explicit, quantitative judgements concerning the prescription of treatment, clinical decision analysis and cost effectiveness analysis. In reporting the results of individual randomized trials as well as meta-analyses of sets of randomized trials, therefore, it should be recognized that the size of

Table 8.5 Treatment effect estimators

		Outcome		Total
		Event	No event	
Exposure	Treated	a	b	n_1
	Control	c	d	n_0
		m_1	m_0	T

Event rate in treated group = a/n_1
Event rate in control group = c/n_0
Relative risk = $\dfrac{a/n_1}{c/n_0}$
Odds ratio = $\dfrac{a/b}{c/d}$
Risk difference = $a/n_1 - c/n_0$
Relative risk reduction = $1 -$ relative risk
Number needed to treat = $1/$risk difference

difference, not just the fact of difference, will have direct implications for clinical practice[26]. The measures of treatment effect which are reported should facilitate their practical application. The risk ratio, or relative risk, is the traditional effect estimator from prospective studies, of which randomized trials are a special case. The estimator provides an answer to the clinically important question: what is the proportion of treated patients, relative to control patients, who experience an event? Its complement, relative risk reduction, provides an answer to a second clinically important question: by how much, in relative terms, is the event rate reduced? The risk difference provides an answer to a third clinically important question: what is the absolute difference in event rate between the treated and control groups? Its inverse, number needed to treat (NNT), provides an answer to a fourth clinically important question: how many patients does one need to treat to expect to prevent one patient experiencing an event?

Each of these estimators can be used to express the effect of treatment in an analysis of a single trial or the typical effect of treatment in a 'meta-analysis' of a set of comparable trials. In meta-analyses, the odds ratio has been used most frequently. Despite the popularity of odds ratio as an effect estimator in meta-analysis, it suffers from the fact that it does not directly address a clinically important question concerning size of treatment effect. However, when the incidence of the event in the control group (i.e. the pretreatment risk) is known, the odds ratio can be converted to the clinically more meaningful risk ratio:

$$\text{Risk ratio} = \frac{\text{OR}}{1 + \text{PR (OR} - 1)}$$

where OR = odds ratio
       PR = pretreatment risk.

Statistical methods. Statistical methods are available for computing each of the various estimators of treatment effect and its confidence interval, both for individual trials and for typical estimators across a set of trials[27,28]. The typical effect is a weighted average, the weights being the inverse of the variance of the estimate provided by each participating trial.

These methods are based on either fixed effect or random effect models[28,29]. Using a fixed effect model, inference is based on the trials actually done, whereas with a random effects model, inference is based on the assumption that the actual trials represent a hypothetical population of trials. Using the fixed effect model, the overall result is not directly influenced by heterogeneity among the effects of treatment in different trials, whereas the random effects model assumes statistical heterogeneity and incorporates it into the estimate of effect. As a result, confidence intervals around treatment effect are usually somewhat wider for analyses based on the random effects model[28].

Heterogeneity in this context refers to the variation in results among the trials contributing to the meta-analysis. The issue of heterogeneity can be considered from both a clinical and statistical perspective: are the differences in results among trials clinically important, and are they unlikely to have arisen by chance? In a meta-analysis of a set of trials having small or moderate sample size, clinically important heterogeneity of results may not be statistically significant. Conversely, among a set of large trials, clinically unimportant heterogeneity may be statistically significant.

Heterogeneity that is both clinically important and statistically significant should trigger consideration of its source, e.g. differences between trials in their clinical features (patient characteristics at entry, intensity or duration of treatment, definition or measurement of outcomes) or in their methodological quality.

Subgroup analyses.   Analyses of treatment effect by subgroups may conform to a priori questions or may be exploratory, hypothesis generating activities. As a general rule, the results of subgroup analyses, even though they may be clinically interesting, should be distrusted[30,31] unless they meet the criteria listed in Table 8.6.

Sensitivity analysis.   Analyses may be undertaken to determine the robustness of the results to variation among trials in one or more important features. Mention has already been made of the use of trial quality scores in this regard. Similarly, the results of the meta-analysis may be examined to determine their sensitivity to important

Table 8.6 Subgroup analyses

---

1. Specify hypothesis-testing subgroup analyses a priori, and limit their number
2. Interpret subgroup analyses cautiously
    distinguish whether protocol driven or data driven
    consider whether supported by plausible causal mechanisms
    examine for consistency across studies
    determine whether statistically significant after adjustment for multiple testing

---

Adapted from Cook et al[5].

assumptions or decisions in conducting the systematic review, e.g. whether unpublished trials are included or excluded.

Inferences Based on Systematic Reviews

The strength of inference derivable from a systematic review depends first of all on the methodological quality of the primary studies on which the review was based. A set of randomized trials of high quality provides a basis for strong inference concerning the probable benefits and risk of treatment. Secondly, strength of inference depends on the degree of consistency of results among the studies reviewed. A set of trials that are consistent in their results (i.e. no clinically or statistically important heterogeneity) allows strong inference concerning probable treatment effects. Thirdly, assurance that the body of research contributing to the review is comprehensive (i.e. exhaustive search strategy and no evidence of publication bias) leads to a basis for strong inference.

Answers to two questions are wanted concerning the efficacy and safety of treatment: is the treatment effect real (i.e. not due to chance, statistically significant), and what is the size of treatment effect? Meta-analysis has the potential to provide valid and precise answers to each of these questions. The statistical significance of a treatment effect is demonstrated when the confidence interval around the point estimate of treatment effect excludes 'no difference'; this would occur when the confidence interval of the typical estimate for relative risk or odds ratio does not include one, or when the confidence interval of the typical estimate for absolute risk reduction does not include zero.

The clinical significance of a treatment effect begs consideration of the size of treatment effect in relation to treatment side effects and economic costs. For a treatment to be recommended, it must be clear that its use would lead to benefits that outweigh harm. Thus, a clinically meaningful way of expressing the result of a trial (or of a meta-analysis of a set of trials) is to report the number of patients one needs to treat (NNT) to expect to prevent one patient having the adverse target event. NNT is calculated as the inverse of the absolute risk reduction caused by treatment. When, as is frequently the case, relative risk reduction is fairly constant over the range of baseline risk, then NNT will necessarily vary, being high at low baseline risk and low at high baseline risk. Toxicity of treatment must be weighed against NNT in order to make a treatment recommendation. Thus, at high baseline risk where NNT is low, a treatment is more likely to be justified than at low baseline risk where NNT is high. Thus, baseline risk is a necessary element to be considered in making a treatment recommendation.

SYSTEMATIC REVIEW OF EFFECT OF ANTENATAL CORTICOSTEROID ON INCIDENCE OF RESPIRATORY DISTRESS SYNDROME AND NEONATAL DEATH

The principles discussed above will now be applied to an important clinical issue – the efficacy of antenatal corticosteroid for the prevention of respiratory distress syndrome (RDS) and neonatal death. A systematic review of randomized trials that have addressed this issue has been conducted by Crowley[32,33]. The most recent update of this review[32] included the results of 18 trials, 15 of which provided information on the incidence of RDS and randomized a total of 3438 fetuses. Fourteen trials reported the incidence of neonatal death. The data extracted by Crowley from these trials are shown in Tables 8.7 and 8.8. These data will be used in the following discussion.

The Oxford Database of Perinatal Trials[12,13] was used by Crowley to identify all relevant trials, both published and, as far as could be

Table 8.7 Effect of antenatal corticosteroid on incidence of respiratory distress syndrome

Trial	Year	No. with RDS/No. randomized	
		Treatment	Control
Liggins	1972	49/532	84/538
Block	1977	5/69	12/61
Morrison	1978	6/67	14/59
Taeusch	1979	7/56	14/71
Papageorgiou	1979	7/71	23/75
Doran	1980	4/81	10/63
Schutte	1980	11/64	17/58
Teramo	1980	3/38	3/42
US Collaborative	1981	42/371	59/372
Schmidt	1984	9/34	10/31
Morales	1986	30/121	63/124
Gamsu	1989	7/131	16/137
Carlen	1991	1/11	4/13
Garite	1992	21/40	28/42
Eronen	1993	13/29	16/37

Data are those used by Crowley[32] for meta-analysis.

Table 8.8 Effect of antenatal corticosteroid on incidence of neonatal death

Trial	Year	Neonatal death/No. randomized	
		Treatment	Control
Liggins	1972	36/532	60/538
Block	1977	1/69	5/61
Morrison	1978	2/67	7/59
Taeusch	1979	5/56	7/71
Papageorgiou	1979	1/71	5/75
Doran	1980	2/81	10/63
Schutte	1980	3/64	12/58
Teramo	1980	0/38	0/42
US Collaborative	1981	36/371	37/372
Schmidt	1984	5/34	5/31
Morales	1986	7/121	13/124
Gamsu	1989	14/131	20/137
Garite	1992	9/40	11/41
Eronen	1993	3/29	2/37

Data are those utilized by Crowley[32] for meta-analysis.

ascertained, unpublished. The quality of each trial was systematically evaluated for three characteristics: blinding of randomization, whether primary analyses were based on all patients randomized, and blinding of outcome measurements. Of these three criteria, the one considered by Crowley to be most important was the control of selection bias at entry by the care taken to blind the randomization.

A fixed effect model was assumed by Crowley in the meta-analysis of results. No statistical heterogeneity was detected with respect to the effect of antenatal corticosteroid on RDS or neonatal death.

The evidence from these 15 trials concerning the effect of antenatal corticosteroid on RDS is shown graphically in Figure 8.1. For each trial, the absolute risk difference and its 95% confidence interval is shown. In 6 of the 15 trials, there was a statistically significant reduction in the incidence of RDS (as shown by the fact that the 95% CI bar does not cross zero). Overall, there is a reduction in the incidence of RDS that is highly statistically significant: absolute risk difference −7.9% (95% CI −5.6%, −10.2%). Table 8.9 uses various treatment effect estimators to express the efficacy of antenatal corticosteroid in reducing the incidence of RDS. Note the typical estimate for relative risk reduction, 41%; absolute risk reduction, 7.9%; NNT, 13. The 95% confidence intervals are given for each.

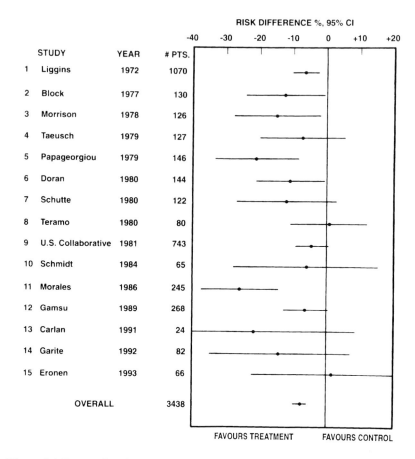

Figure 8.1 Conventional meta-analysis of trials testing the effect of antenatal corticosteroid on incidence of RDS. Data are taken from the trials included in the meta-analysis of Crowley[32]. Treatment effect, expressed as risk difference, is shown for each trial as the point estimate and 95% confidence interval. If the 95% CI does not cross zero, the effect is statistically significant ($P < 0.05$) in that trial. Six of 15 trials showed a statistically significant reduction in RDS, whereas each of the other nine trials failed to demonstrate a statistically significant effect. The typical estimate, overall, is that this set of trials shows a reduction in incidence of RDS that is statistically highly significant.

Assuming constant relative risk reduction one can calculate the absolute risk reduction over a range of baseline risks for RDS, and the corresponding NNT. These results are given in Figure 8.2. It is clearly evident that the number of fetuses that need to be treated with

Table 8.9 Effect of corticosteroid prior to preterm delivery on respiratory distress syndrome, overall

	Point estimate	95% CI
Relative risk reduction (%)	−41	−32, −49
Absolute risk reduction (%)	−7.9	−5.6, −10.2
Number needed to treat	13	10, 18

Calculated from meta-analysis of Crowley (15 trials, 588 events, 3438 subjects).

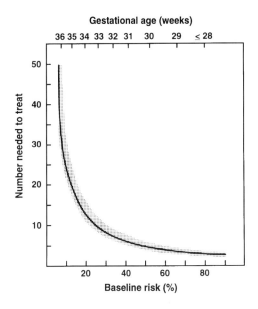

Figure 8.2 Number of fetuses that need to be treated with antenatal corticosteroid to prevent one case of RDS, as a function of baseline risk. Number needed to treat is derived from the typical relative risk reduction of 41% calculated from the data of the trials included in the meta-analysis of Crowley[32]. The gestational ages corresponding to baseline risk are based on the data of Usher et al[34]. Shaded zone indicates 95% confidence interval.

antenatal corticosteroid to expect to prevent one case of RDS varies with baseline risk. At a high baseline risk of ≥50% (corresponding to gestational ages of ≤30 weeks), NNT is low. However, at a low baseline risk of 15% (corresponding to gestational ages above 34 weeks) NNT rises sharply. This phenomenon is explicitly demonstrated by subgroup analyses based on gestational age at randomization. If gestational age is less than 31 weeks, one needs to treat five fetuses in order to prevent one case of RDS (Table 8.10), based on the data from nine trials. If gestational age is more than 34 weeks, one needs to treat 94 fetuses in order to prevent one case of RDS (Table 8.11), based on the data from eight trials. Because the effect in this latter gestational age group is not quite statistically significant, the upper bound of the 95% confidence interval for NNT includes infinity. These data were important determinants of the NIH Consensus Development Panel's recommendation that all fetuses between 24 and 34 weeks gestation should be considered candidates for antenatal corticosteroid treatment[35].

Table 8.10 Effect of corticosteroid prior to preterm delivery on respiratory distress syndrome in babies <31 weeks gestation

	Point estimate	95% CI
Relative risk reduction (%)	−37	−23, −49
Absolute risk reduction (%)	−19	−11, −27
Number needed to treat	5	4, 9

Calculated from meta-analysis of Crowley (9 trials, 203 events, 461 subjects).

Table 8.11 Effect of corticosteroid prior to preterm delivery on respiratory distress syndrome in babies >34 weeks gestation

	Point estimate	95% CI
Relative risk reduction (%)	−37	+29, −69
Absolute risk reduction (%)	−1.1	+ 1.3, −3.4
Number needed to treat	94	30, infinite

Calculated from meta-analysis of Crowley (8 trials, 29 events, 886 subjects).

The evidence from 14 trials concerning the effect of antenatal corticosteroid on neonatal deaths is shown in Figure 8.3 and in Table 8.12. In order to prevent one neonatal death, one needs to expose 22 fetuses to corticosteroid (95% CI 16, 39). Again, this estimate will vary with baseline risk, following the pattern shown in Figure 8.2.

Impact of Systematic Reviews on Planning of Future Trials

One can ask the question: at what point in the history of trials of antenatal corticosteroid for fetal lung maturation was the aggregated

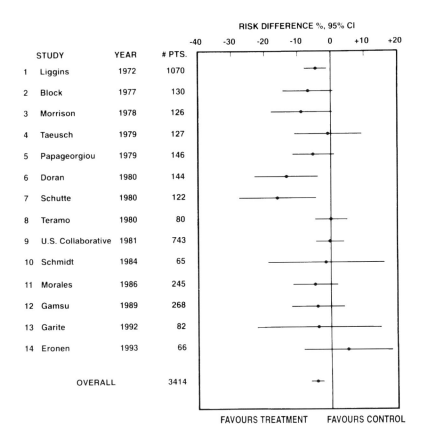

Figure 8.3 Conventional meta-analysis of trials testing the effect of antenatal corticosteroid on incidence of neonatal death. Data are taken from the trials included in the meta-analysis of Crowley[32]. Treatment effect, expressed as risk difference, is shown for each trial as the point estimate and 95% confidence interval. If the 95% CI does not cross zero, the effect is statistically significant (*P* <0.05) in that trial. Three of 14 trials showed a statistically significant reduction in neonatal deaths, whereas each of the other 11 trials failed to demonstrate a statistically significant effect. The typical estimate, overall, is that this set of trials shows a reduction in incidence of RDS that is statistically highly significant.

evidence from randomized trials sufficient to show that this treatment reduces the incidence of RDS and of neonatal death? One can reconstruct the history of the growth of evidence by ordering the trials by their date of publication and performing a new meta-analysis each time a new trial is published – the technique of 'cumulative meta-analysis'[36].

Table 8.12 Effect of corticosteroid prior to preterm delivery
on neonatal deaths

	Point estimate	95% CI
Absolute risk reduction (%)	−4.5	−2.6, −6.4
Number needed to treat	22	16, 39

Calculated from meta-analysis of Crowley (14 trials, 318 events, 3414 subjects).

Figure 8.4 presents the same data as in Figure 8.1 in the form of a cumulative meta-analysis. The reduction in RDS was statistically significant in the first trial and as subsequent trials were reported it has remained so. Moreover, the point estimate for size of effect, expressed as absolute risk reduction, has changed very little with the addition of data from subsequent trials. However, the 95% confidence interval has narrowed, indicating increased precision of the estimate of effect as subsequent trials were reported. The same data can also be plotted as a time trend of the accumulating evidence that corticosteroid prior to preterm delivery reduces the incidence of RDS (Figure 8.5).

Cumulative meta-analyses (Figures 8.6 and 8.7) are also shown for the effect on neonatal death. The risk reduction for neonatal death was statistically significant in the first trial and has remained so as each subsequent trial is added to the cumulative meta-analysis. The point estimate for the size of effect, expressed as absolute risk reduction and as NNT, has changed very little since the reports of the first trial, but the precision of the estimate has increased over time.

Thus, cumulative meta-analysis demonstrates that we have known since 1972, and with a high degree of confidence, that antenatal corticosteroid reduces the incidence of RDS and of neonatal death. One wonders whether cumulative meta-analysis of the results of previous trials, had it been available, would have persuaded against the launching of some of the later placebo controlled trials testing the efficacy of antenatal corticosteroid in preventing RDS.

Thus, the conduct of a systematic review provides a sound basis for identifying the most important hypotheses to be tested in a new trial. An up to date, systematic review can show whether a new trial of a previously tested therapy is in fact needed and, if so, why. The design of a new trial will be determined by the result of the systematic review of previous trials: in whom should the treatment now be tested, against what alternative, and with what outcomes? The required sample size of a trial is traditionally calculated as that needed to identify a clinically important treatment effect if it is pres-

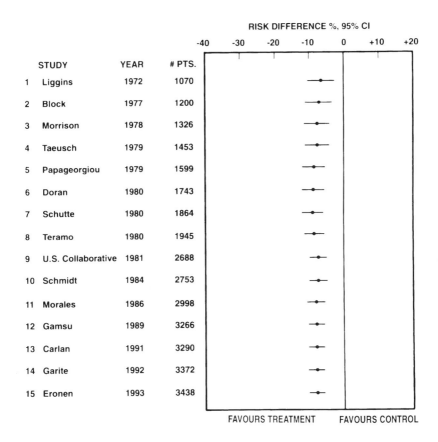

Figure 8.4 Cumulative meta-analysis of trials testing the effect of antenatal corticosteroid on incidence of RDS. Data are taken from the trials included in the meta-analysis of Crowley[32]. Treatment effect, expressed as risk difference, is shown as in Figure 8.1 except that the meta-analysis is repeated each time a new trial is published. The effect was statistically significant in the first trial (Liggins 1972) and has remained so since. The point estimate for the size of effect expressed as risk difference has changed very little since the reports of the first trial. However, subsequent trials have added increasing precision to the estimate of effect, indicated by the narrowing of the 95% CI.

ent, as if no prior trials of the same treatment had been performed[37]. In future, we may see trials having a sample size calculated as sufficient to overturn the results of the existing systematic review of all previous trials (for example, sufficient to change a 'no difference' result to a statistically significant result). Systematic reviews of previous trials, including as they do a review of methodological quality,

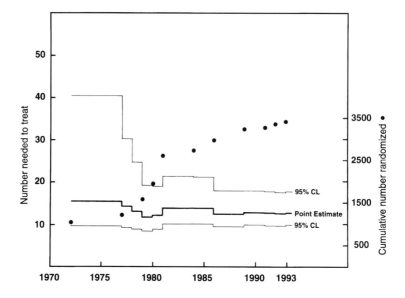

Figure 8.5 Time trend of accumulating evidence that corticosteroid prior to preterm delivery reduces the incidence of RDS. The effect was statistically significant in the first trial (1972) and has remained so since. The point estimate for the size of effect, expressed as number needed to treat, has changed very little since the reports of the first trial. However, subsequent trials have added increasing precision to the estimate of effect, indicated by the narrowing of the 95% confidence limits (95% CL) over time. Number needed to treat is calculated from the absolute risk reduction in the trials reviewed by Crowley[32].

will often identify methodological weaknesses of prior trials and suggest opportunities for improvements in the design, conduct or reporting of future trials.

Evidence based Practice of Neonatology/Perinatology

Despite the evidence of efficacy in reducing RDS and death rates, the use by obstetricians of antenatal corticosteroid has remained low by many accounts. For example, in the Canadian multicentre trial of ritodrine for preterm labour, corticosteroid was used in only 35 and 36% of the treatment and control groups respectively. The practice of evidence based neonatology/perinatology[38] would be fostered by the more ready availability of up to date evidence in the form of systematic reviews of results of randomized trials.

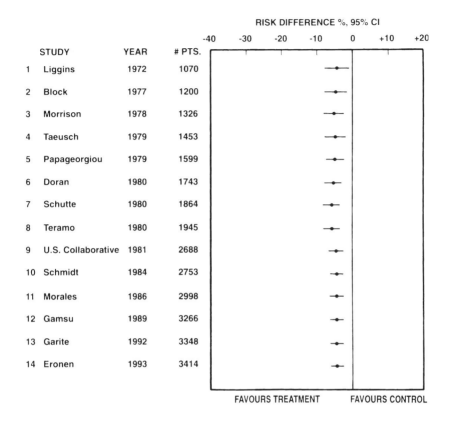

Figure 8.6 Cumulative meta-analysis of trials testing the effect of antenatal corticosteroid on incidence of neonatal death. Data are taken from the trials included in the meta-analysis of Crowley[32]. Treatment effect, expressed as risk difference, is shown as in Figure 8.3 except that the meta-analysis is repeated each time a new trial is published. The effect was statistically significant in the first trial (Liggins 1972) and has remained so since. The point estimate for the size of effect expressed as risk difference has changed very little since the reports of the first trial. However, subsequent trials have added increasing precision to the estimate of effect, indicated by the narrowing of the 95% confidence interval.

A project to register all reports of randomized trials in neonatology/perinatology was undertaken by Iain Chalmers and his colleagues at the UK National Perinatal Epidemiology Unit[12]. The result, the Oxford Database of Perinatal Trials, provided the database for systematic reviews of evidence of efficacy and safety of treatments in perinatology[39,40] and neonatology[19]. There is now underway, under

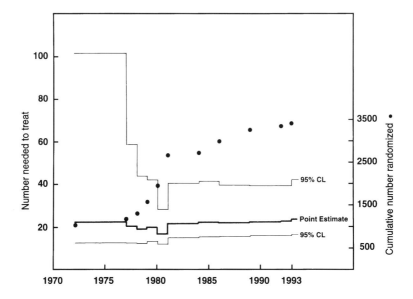

Figure 8.7 Time trend of accumulating evidence that corticosteroid prior to preterm delivery reduces the incidence of neonatal death. The effect was statistically significant in the first trial (1972) and has remained so since. The point estimate for the size of effect, expressed as number needed to treat, has changed very little since the reports of the first trial. However, subsequent trials have added increased precision to the estimate of effect indicated by the narrowing of the 95% confidence limits (95% CL) over time. Number needed to treat is calculated from the absolute risk reduction in the trials reviewed by Crowley[32].

the aegis of the Cochrane Collaboration, an international effort not only in perinatology[41,42] but across all fields of medicine to review systematically and quantitatively the evidence from randomized trials and to make the results available in the form of periodically up dated systematic reviews incorporating meta-analyses[43]. As part of this effort, the Neonatal Collaborative Review Group of the Cochrane Collaboration plans to update periodically the reviews contained in *Effective Care of the Newborn Infant*[19]. A specialized database, the Cochrane Neonatal Database, will be published electronically and revised at frequent intervals as new evidence from neonatal trials becomes available.

The task of implementing evidence based care depends first, but not only, on identifying what works and what does not; systematic reviews of evidence are a necessary but not sufficient contributor to evidence based practice[42]. The identification and evaluation of methods to promote the adoption in neonatal/perinatal clinical practice of evidence based treatment recommendation will be in itself a research challenge[44].

REFERENCES

1. Mulrow CD. The medical review article: state of the science. *Ann Intern Med* 1987;**106:**485–488.
2. Sacks HS, Berrier J, Reitman D et al. Meta-analysis of randomized controlled trials. *N Engl J Med* 1987;**316:**450–455.
3. Antman EM, Lau J, Kupelnick B et al. A comparison of results of meta-analysis of randomized control trials and recommendations of clinical experts. *JAMA* 1992;**268:**240–248.
4. Peto R. Why do we need systematic overviews of randomized trials? *Stat Med* 1987;**6:**233–240.
5. Cook DJ, Sackett DL and Spitzer WO. Methodologic guidelines for systematic reviews of randomized control trials in health care from the Potsdam Consultation on meta-analysis. *J Clin Epidemiol* 1995;**48:**167–171.
6. Kirpalani H, Schmidt B, McKibbon KA et al. Searching MEDLINE for randomized clinical trials involving care of the newborn. *Pediatrics* 1989;**83:**543–546.
7. Haynes RB, Wilczynski N, McKibbon KA et al. Developing optimal search strategies for detecting clinically sound studies in MEDLINE. *J Am Informatics Assoc* 1994;**1:**447–458.
8. Koren G, Shear H, Graham K and Einarson T. Bias against the null hypothesis: the reproductive hazards of cocaine. *Lancet* 1989;**ii:**1440–1442.
9. Dickersin K, Min Y and Meinert CL. Factors influencing publication of research results. *JAMA* 1992;**267:**374–378.
10. Easterbrook PJ, Berlin JA, Gopalan R and Matthews DR. Publication bias in clinical research. *Lancet* 1991;**337:**867–872.
11. Cook DJ, Guyatt GH, Ryan G et al. Should unpublished data be included in meta-analyses? Current conviction and controversies. *JAMA* 1993; **269:**2749–2753.
12. Chalmers I, Hetherington J, Newdick M et al. The Oxford Database of Perinatal Trials: developing a register of published reports of controlled trials. *Controlled Clin Trials* 1986;**7:**306–324.
13. Hetherington J, Dickersin K, Chalmers I and Meinert CL. Retrospective and prospective identification of unpublished controlled trials: lessons from a survey of obstetricians and pediatricians. *Pediatrics* 1989;**84:**374–380.
14. Sacks H, Chalmers TC and Smith H. Randomized versus historical controls for clinical trials. *Am J Med* 1982;**72:**233–240.
15. Chalmers TC, Celani P, Sacks HS and Smith H. Bias in treatment assignment in controlled clinical trials. *N Engl J Med* 1983;**309:**1358–1361.

16. Gray-Donald K and Kramer MS. Causality inference in observational vs experimental studies. An empirical comparison. *Am J Epidemiol* 1988;**127**:885–892.

17. Chalmers TC, Smith H, Blackburn B et al. A method for assessing the quality of a randomized controlled trial. *Controlled Clin Trials* 1981;**2**:31–49.

18. Reisch JS, Tyson JE and Mize SG. Aid to the evaluation of therapeutic studies. *Pediatrics* 1989;**84**:815–827.

19. Sinclair JC and Bracken MB (eds). *Effective Care of the Newborn Infant.* Oxford: Oxford University Press, 1992.

20. Tyson JE, Furzan JA, Reisch JS and Mize SG. An evaluation of the quality of therapeutic studies in perinatal medicine. *J Pediatr* 1983;**102**:10–13.

21. Schulz KF, Chalmers I, Grimes DA and Altman DG. Assessing the quality of randomization from reports of controlled trials published in obstetrics and gynecology journals. *JAMA* 1994;**272**:125–128.

22. Williams DH and Davis CE. Reporting of assignment methods in clinical trials. *Controlled Clin Trials* 1994;**15**:294–298.

23. The Standards of Reporting Trials Group. A proposal for structured reporting of randomized controlled trials. *JAMA* 1994;**272**:1926–1931.

24. Working Group on Recommendations for Reporting of Clinical Trials in the Biomedical Literature. Call for comments on a proposal to improve reporting of clinical trials in the biomedical literature. *Ann Intern Med* 1994;**121**:894–895.

25. Detsky AS, Naylor CD, O'Rourke K et al. Incorporating variations in the quality of individual randomized trials into meta-analysis. *J Clin Epidemiol* 1992;**45**:255–265.

26. Sinclair JC and Bracken MB. Clinically useful measures of effect in binary analyses of randomized trials. *J Clin Epidemiol* 1994;**47**:881–889.

27. Bracken MB. Statistical methods for analysis of effect of treatment in overviews of randomized trials. In: Sinclair JC and Bracken MB (eds) *Effective Care of the Newborn Infant.* Oxford: Oxford University Press, 1992: 13–18.

28. Fleiss JL. The statistical basis of meta-analysis. *Stat Meth Med Res* 1993;**2**:121–145.

29. DerSimonian R and Laird N. Meta-analysis in clinical trials. *Controlled Clin Trials* 1986;**7**:177–188.

30. Yusuf S, Wittes J, Probstfiel J and Tyroler HA. Analysis and interpretation of treatment effects in subgroups of patients in randomized clinical trials. *JAMA* 1991;**266**:93–98.

31. Oxman AD and Guyatt GH. A consumers guide to subgroup analyses. *Ann Intern Med* 1992;**116**:78–84.

32. Crowley PA. Antenatal corticosteroid therapy: A meta-analysis of the randomized trials, 1972 to 1994. *Am J Obstet Gynecol* 1995;**173**:322–335.

33. Crowley P. Corticosteroids prior to preterm delivery. In: Enkin MW, Keirse MJNC, Renfrew MJ and Neilson JP (eds). *Pregnancy and Childbirth Module.* Cochrane Database of Systematic Reviews: Review No. 2955, 26 April 1993. Published through Cochrane Updates on Disk, Oxford. Update Software, Spring 1993.

34. Usher RH, Allen AC and McLean FH. Risk of respiratory distress syndrome related to gestational age, route of delivery, and maternal diabetes. *Am J Obstet Gynecol* 1971;**111:**826–832.

35. NIH Consensus Development Panel on the Effect of Corticosteroids for Fetal Maturation on Perinatal Outcomes. Effect of corticosteroids for fetal maturation on perinatal outcomes. *JAMA* 1995;**273:**413–418.

36. Lau J, Antman EM, Jimenez-Silva J, Kupelnick B, Mosteller F and Chalmers TC. Cumulative meta-analysis of therapeutic trials for myocardial infarction. *N Engl J Med* 1992;**327:**248–254.

37. Chalmers TC. Meta-analytic stimulus for changes in clinical trials. *Stat Methods Med Res* 1993;**2:**161–172.

38. Evidence-Based Medicine Working Group. Evidence-based medicine. A new approach to teaching the practice of medicine. *JAMA* 1992; **268:**2420–2425.

39. Chalmers I, Enkin MW and Keirse MJNC (eds). *Effective Care in Pregnancy and Childbirth*. Oxford: Oxford University Press, 1989.

40. Chalmers I, Enkin MW and Keirse MJNC. Preparing and updating systematic reviews of randomized controlled trials of health care. *Milbank Q* 1993;**71:**411–437.

41. Cochrane Collaboration. *Cochrane Pregnancy and Childbirth Database.* Oxford: Update Software, 1993.

42. Enkin MW. Systematic summaries and dissemination of evidence: The Cochrane Pregnancy and Childbirth Database. *Semin Perinatol* 1995;**19:** 155–160.

43. Chalmers I. The Cochrane Collaboration: preparing, maintaining and disseminating systematic reviews of the effects of health care. *Ann NY Acad Sci* 1993;**703:**156–163.

44. Lomas J, Enkin MW, Anderson GM et al. Opinion leaders vs audit and feedback to implement practice guidelines. *JAMA* 1991;**265:**2202–2207.

9

What Causes Neonatal Necrotizing Enterocolitis and How can it be Prevented?

David A. Clark and Mark J.S. Miller

INTRODUCTION

Neonatal necrotizing enterocolitis (NEC) is an overwhelming gastro-intestinal illness of preterm infants, afflicting 5–30% of babies born weighing less than 1500 g. Causation theories have included hypoxic-ischaemic mucosal injury, the 'undiscovered organism' and specific inflammatory mediators[1]. The disease has caused considerable confusion and discussion because, theoretically, all preterm infants are susceptible. In many situations, a preterm infant has no known predisposing factor yet develops devastating disease. Alternatively, infants may possess a multitude of 'predisposing factors' but do not display gastrointestinal illness. Additionally, even the earliest clinical signs indicate advanced gastrointestinal disease. Thus, initiating events may pass without recognition or intervention.

Over 90% of infants with necrotizing enterocolitis are born at less than 34 weeks gestation and most of these have been enterally fed[2]. Prematurity and feedings provide the only two associations that are firmly established with necrotizing enterocolitis. However, a very disturbing report from the National Institute of Child Health and Development (NICHD) Neonatal Network revealed a variation in NEC prevalence from as low as 3.9% to a peak of 22.4% of infants less than 1500 g[3]. In this study 'intercenter differences were the most significant factor in determining NEC prevalence'. No other illness in this study group, including patent ductus arteriosus, intraventricular haemorrhage and respiratory distress, were significantly different from one facility to another. This strongly suggests that clinical practices within a facility determine the risk of necrotizing enterocolitis in comparable preterm infants; in simpler terms, NEC has an iatrogenic component.

Necrotizing enterocolitis is not a disease from a single aetiology but rather is 'end stage intestinal pathology' which may have derived from any one of several initial insults. Further, it may represent a family of diseases with distinct initiating events that culminate in severe intestinal damage. This chapter will examine the epidemiological information and attempt to place it in the context of current clinical and animal research. The focus will be on the initiation of injury, whether intrinsic or extrinsic, and the propagation of the intestinal damage.

CLINICAL STUDIES OF EPIDEMIOLOGY

Reports that include all cases of necrotizing enterocolitis within a particular facility are somewhat confusing in that often they summarize all babies without differentiating gestational age, birthweight, perinatal asphyxia, hypoxic-ischaemic 'risk factors', the time of onset of disease, or feeding (quantity or type). In most reports, infants greater than 36 weeks gestation who develop 'NEC' have either perinatal asphyxia, or intestinal motility is profoundly disturbed (e.g. Hirschsprung disease)[4]. In the case of perinatal asphyxia, the intestinal illness presents as a portion of a multiorgan system failure. In Hirschsprung disease, it is initiated within the intestine but may rapidly progress to systemic complications. In the absence of one of these risk factors, necrotizing enterocolitis in a fullterm infant is rare.

The time of onset of NEC in term babies is shortly after birth. Thilo et al reported a mean gestational age of 37.9 ± 2 weeks in 13 babies who developed NEC in the first day of life, compared with 66 preterm babies (gestational age 32.0 ± 3.5 weeks) who developed NEC after 1 day of age[5]. deGamarra et al[4] and Andrews et al[6] reported term infants who presented with signs and symptoms of NEC by 7 days of age, most of whom had not been fed. The median age of onset of NEC in 43 fullterm infants was 2 days, with 42% presenting in the first day of life.

Stoll et al, using a multiple regression analysis case–control study of 32 cases of NEC and 95 controls, reported that Apgar scores, respiratory distress and hypotension did *not* correlate with the initiation of necrotizing enterocolitis[7]. The risk of developing necrotizing enterocolitis was inversely related to gestational age and birthweight; the smaller preterm infants were at greatest risk. Prematurity remains a prime risk factor, but the time of onset of NEC is usually weeks after birth.

The National Collaborative NICHD Study of patent ductus arteriosus[8] confirmed the association of low birthweight with necrotizing enterocolitis. Additionally, the study demonstrated that NEC is *not* readily associated with perinatal asphyxia or respiratory distress syndrome, nor the status of systemic circulation, including patency of the ductus arteriosus. The lack of relationship to historical risk factors is not surprising because the majority of the NEC cases were initiated by feeding associated mechanisms and did not result from a cardiovascular insult.

An often overlooked and yet very important study of 129 infants with NEC was reported by Marchildon et al[9]. NEC cases were analysed with respect to fed versus unfed and necrosis (perforation) requiring surgery versus no surgery. The infants who did not require surgery in both the fed and non-fed categories were similar in birthweight, gestational age and Apgar scores. Seven babies who had not been fed and did not have surgery had an average age of onset of NEC of less than 5 days and had multiple risk factors for hypoxic-ischaemic or hypotensive insult. However, the 45 infants who had been fed before the onset of their disease had an average age of onset at 13 days and significantly less respiratory distress, fewer umbilical artery catheters, perinatal asphyxia and patent ductus arteriosus. Similarly, when they examined 77 infants who required surgery, there was a ratio of 1:10 from the non-fed to fed infants. The seven unfed infants were smaller (average birthweight 1000 g). All of these infants had at least one risk factor for significant ischaemic injury to the intestine. In the 70 fed infants who developed intestinal necrosis, the mean age of onset was 14 days with a much lower incidence of risk factors for hypoxic-ischaemic injury to the intestine. Of great importance is the site of necrosis of the intestine. In the babies requiring surgery who had not been fed, the primary site of perforation was the duodenum (43%) and there were no sites of multiple perforation. However, in the infants who had been fed, the distal ileum and the right colon accounted for over 50% of disease and an additional 18% had multiple sites of perforation. This study clearly demonstrates that NEC presents in fed infants at a later time and at different loci than in unfed infants. Only the unfed, early onset form of NEC displayed risk factors for ischaemic injury to the intestine.

In a study of infants of multiple gestation who developed NEC, Samm et al reported that the healthier twin (twin A), with fewer risk factors for ischaemic bowel injury, acquired NEC after being fed more rapidly than the 'sicker' twins[10]. This suggested that feeding rather than cardiovascular risk factors are involved in initiating NEC and perhaps identifies a clinical practice that could determine the baseline incidence of endemic NEC in a neonatal intensive care unit.

The NICHD umbilical artery catheter study revealed no difference in the incidence of NEC with a high versus a low umbilical arterial catheter[11]. Two per cent of infants in each group had onset of NEC in the first 6 days of life. Only these babies had significant perinatal hypotension requiring volume expansion compared with unaffected babies. In contrast, there was a sevenfold increase in the incidence of NEC from 1 week to 3 months of age in both high and low catheter groups and no correlation with perinatal ischaemic risk factors.

Although the risk factors for ischaemia–reperfusion injury in the newborn have been aggressively addressed, the incidence of necrotizing enterocolitis has not decreased since 1980. Ischaemia–reperfusion injury initiates only a small fraction of NEC cases. We postulate that NEC (inflammatory bowel disease) following feeding is the most common aetiology. It is more severe and afflicts primarily the preterm infant born weighing less than 1500 g. Table 9.1 summarizes the epidemiology of endemic NEC in infants by feeding status[2–19].

Table 9.1 Associations of NEC and feeding

	Unfed infant	Fed infant
Gestational age	Preterm to term	<34 weeks
Birthweight	All	<1500 g
Perinatal asphyxia	Common	Less likely
Bacterial colonization	Little	Well established 3–5 days after feedings
Onset of NEC	<7 days after birth	6 days–3 months (25% >1 month)
Location of necrosis	Small bowel; single site	Ileum/colon; multiple sites common
Organ system involvement	Multiple (brain, kidneys, heart)	Initially intestine, then systemic
Evidence of pre-existing intestinal dysfunction	Minimal	Carbohydrate malabsorption; poor motility; decreased stools

INFECTIOUS AETIOLOGY OF NEC

Most cases of necrotizing enterocolitis occur sporadically. However, necrotizing enterocolitis may occur in clusters, which are usually super-imposed upon the baseline rate, suggesting an additional infectious com-ponent at these times[20]. During these epidemics, the infants afflicted with NEC have higher birthweights with fewer perinatal complications. Concurrently, it is common to have an increased frequency of gastro-intestinal illness among the intensive care nursery staff, and other infants commonly have gastrointestinal symptoms, including diarrhoea.

A wide variety of infectious agents have been associated with necrotizing enterocolitis (Table 9.2)[20,21]. In the few reports in which enteropathogens have been identified in outbreaks, diarrhoea was the most common presentation and necrotizing enterocolitis developed in only a few of these infants. The diarrhoea which occurred in these infants was usually bloody. The feedings were stopped, antibiotics were begun and isolation measures were instituted. The outcome of these afflicted infants is much better than that of the more preterm infants with severe disease.

An important association reported by Carbonaro et al was that organisms isolated from children with necrotizing enterocolitis were capable of more rapid fermentation of carbohydrate[22]. That study demonstrated that a strain of *Klebsiella* segregated into slow and rapid lactose fermentors. When tested in an animal model, only the rapid lactose fermentor strain of *Klebsiella* incubated with half strength premature formula in vivo resulted in intestinal necrosis. The slow fermenting strain of the same *Klebsiella* species in the *same*

Table 9.2 Infectious agents associated with NEC

Bacteria	Viruses
Clostridium butyricum	Coronavirus*
*Clostridium difficile**	Enterovirus
Clostridium perfringens	Rotavirus*
Enterobacter spp.	
*Escherichia coli**	
Klebsiella spp.	
Pseudomonas aeruginosa	
Salmonella spp.*	
Staphylococcus aureus	
Staphylococcus – coagulase negative*	

*Enteropathogenic or toxin producing.

animals produced no intestinal pathology. In addition, the slow fermenting strain of *Klebsiella* could be induced to ferment lactose rapidly by exposure to low dose ampicillin or to tryptone agar, a pancreatic digest of bovine casein. This work emphasizes that the common intestinal flora may play a critical role in generating one of the known intestinal barrier breakers, organic acids. The gaseous products of fermentation, carbon dioxide and hydrogen contribute to pneumatosis intestinalis, an important diagnostic criteria of NEC.

In summary, no single organism has been found to be the cause of necrotizing enterocolitis[23]. Infants with early onset disease have had little time to colonize their intestine and they rarely have been fed. Epidemic NEC, presumed to be infectious agent related, accounts for only approximately 5% of all cases of necrotizing enterocolitis.

PREMATURITY AND NEC

Table 9.3 identifies intestinal risk factors for necrotizing enterocolitis in premature infants. Poor intestinal motility has been well documented in premature infants[24]. The suck–swallow mechanism does not mature until approximately 34 weeks gestation and gastric emptying is delayed. Small intestinal motor activity and colonic function are immature compared with fullterm infants. The neural and hormonal modulation of gastrointestinal motor activity is poorly defined in premature infants. Delayed intestinal transit permits bacterial overgrowth and impairs the clearance of products of fermentation, which could cause intestinal mucosal disruption. Ileus may also result from the intestinal inflammation resulting in neuronal injury, thus reinforcing the problem[25].

A second well defined risk factor for intestinal disease in preterm infants is malabsorption. Much evidence exists for carbohydrate intol-

Table 9.3 Intestinal risk factors – preterm infants

- Poor intestinal motility
- Malabsorption
  Carbohydrate
  Protein
  Lipid
- Intestinal flora
- Immature mucosal defences
- Epithelial permeability

erance and necrotizing enterocolitis[14,17–19,26]. The fermentation of undigested carbohydrate (especially lactose) results in short chain fatty acids (organic acids) and gases (hydrogen and carbon dioxide)[17,19,27]. Positive reducing substances in stool and excess breath hydrogen confirm the malabsorption and intraluminal fermentation. Garcia et al demonstrated excess urinary D-lactate in the urine of infants during the acute phase of necrotizing enterocolitis[28]. Some of these organic acids may be cleared by absorption and urinary excretion. Accumulation of organic acids in the intestinal tract beyond the buffering capacity of mucosal and dietary proteins leads to mucosal disruption.

Once the barrier is broken, inflammation may be readily established by luminal contents, including proteins or protein subunits in the intestinal lumen. The α fraction of bovine casein, which is less well digested by preterm infants, may initiate inflammation by activating mast cells and has been shown to be chemotactic for neutrophils[29,30]. The bacteria, their toxins, or protein derivatives (e.g. formyl-methionyl-leucyl-phenylalanine (fMLP) are also capable of provoking a profound inflammatory response.

Although fat malabsorption is well documented in premature infants, no specific association with fat malabsorption has been found in neonates with NEC. In a piglet model, the combination of intraluminal fats with a significant ischaemic insult results in intestinal inflammation and destruction within the first 48 hours after birth[31]. Beyond this time no similar effect could be shown.

The role of intestinal flora is discussed under infectious aetiologies of NEC. The common intestinal flora, especially in concert with an immature intestinal mucosa and immune defence systems, may be all that is necessary for the initiation of inflammatory bowel disease[17,19,22].

Preterm infants are at greater risk of contracting NEC if they are formula fed and feedings are rapidly advanced. From the previous discussion it is readily seen how excess feedings could overwhelm gut homeostatis in the preterm infant. The composition of formulae for preterm infants is very different from breast milk[32]. Many factors in breast milk, e.g. epidermal growth factor and prostaglandins, enhance mucosal development. The cellular components, secretory IgA, the bifidus factor and lactoferrin all modulate gut microflora.

INITIATION AND PROPAGATION

Numerous agents have been shown to disrupt the intestinal mucosal barrier in humans and animal models. Only four of the agents listed in Table 9.4 are plausible entities as initiators of intestinal injury which progresses to NEC. Ischaemia–reperfusion injury is most common in the unfed infant but cannot be supported as the initiator of epithelial barrier dysfunction in the feeding-associated form of NEC[33]. Bacterial and possibly viral enteropathic organisms contribute to the infrequent epidemic form of necrotizing enterocolitis[20]. The precise nature of this contribution may vary from epidemic to epidemic. Some outbreaks may involve a specific toxin (e.g. staph Δ toxin)[34]. An extensive search has failed to define a toxin or toxins as the cause of feeding induced NEC. In the fed infant, organic acids, generated by bacterial fermentation of carbohydrate, and lipids are ideal candidates for disruption of the mucosal barrier[19,31].

Table 9.4 Agents shown to disrupt the intestinal mucosal barrier

- Acids – organic, HCl*
- Alcohol
- Alkali
- Aspirin
- Bacterial toxins/fMLP*
- Bile salts
- Formaldehyde
- Ischaemia–reperfusion*
- Lipids*
- Non-steroidal anti-inflammatory drugs
- Phorbol ester
- Sulphated polysaccharides

*Potential initiator for neonatal NEC.

The first cell types involved in intestinal injury are those closest to the point of insult. Epithelial cells, mast cells and resident neutrophils are the first line of defence against foreign proteins. Table 9.5 shows the cells and mediators involved in the initiation of the intestinal inflammatory response. These cells release a host of inflammatory mediators and cytokines that lead to the infiltration of blood-borne elements that exacerbate and extend the inflammation[35–37]. It is important to note that the infants with intestinal necrosis from an obvious ischaemic insult (volvulus, aortic thrombosis) have a minimal inflammatory response, which is localized without pneumatosis intestinalis, and normal circulating neutrophils and platelets. The

Table 9.5 Cells and mediators involved in intestinal injury

Initiation	Exacerbation
Epithelial	Neutrophils – recruited
Mast cells	Eosinophils – recruited
Neutrophils – resident	Macrophages
Macrophages	Lymphocytes
Endothelium	Platelets
Inflammatory mediators	
Complement	Oxygen radicals
Endothelin 1	Platelet activating factor
Interleukin 6	Thromboxane
Peptido leukotrienes (C4, D4)	Tumour necrosis factor
Nitric oxide	

infants with feeding associated necrotizing enterocolitis have a much more extensive inflammatory response, commonly with severe neutropenia and thrombocytopenia. The neutropenia and thrombocytopenia cannot be explained by bacteraemia. Only 20–25% of severely affected infants will have bacteraemia. In addition, the bone marrow stores of these infants are not depleted of neutrophils as would be expected in systemic sepsis. Chemotactic mediators released from injured intestine are the most likely source of this systemic response.

A series of mediators are released in the initiation and propagation phases of the intestinal inflammatory response. Endothelin 1, interleukin 6, peptidoleukotrienes, nitric oxide metabolites, platelet activating factor and tumour necrosis factor α (TNF-α) have all been found to be increased in models of NEC and in the serum or urine of infants during the acute phase of necrotizing enterocolitis[35,38,39]. These mediators are released nearly simultaneously and may interact to produce synergistic effects on local circulation and cytotoxicity. The microcirculation may become congested with adherent leucocytes, resulting in decreased perfusion and local oedema. This inflammation negates an important defence mechanism, the clearance of luminal initiators via circulation. A local ischaemic event from a luminal insult is now a well recognized mechanism in gastric ulceration. This would explain the observation that intravenous superoxide dismutase prevents intestinal injury from luminal organic acids[40].

PREVENTION OF NECROTIZING ENTEROCOLITIS

Approximately 10% of infants with NEC develop intestinal necrosis as a result of perinatal ischaemic events. Aggressive obstetric care and prevention of perinatal asphyxia, as well as prompt correction of shock, hypotension and acidosis, may decrease the absolute numbers of this form of NEC.

Infection control measures (e.g. cohorting) may limit the extent of epidemic necrotizing enterocolitis[41]. Since many different organisms have been implicated in epidemic NEC, oral prophylactic antibiotics will not prevent NEC. An uncommon and restricted use of oral antibiotics is appropriate when a specific bacterial toxin (staph Δ toxin) is identified as the causative agent. Oral antibiotics may be useful in infants colonized with the organism to prevent *epidemic* NEC[34]. Antibiotics modify intestinal microflora, but also promote resistant strains. Oral aminoglycosides are absorbed from the immature intestine and achieve ototoxic serum levels. Any single oral antibiotic regimen may actually enhance bacterial carbohydrate fermentation, generating excess organic acids. Therefore indiscriminate use of antibiotics may predispose infants to NEC rather than reduce the risk. Although broad spectrum antibiotics should be administered intravenously once NEC presents clinically, oral antibiotics should not be used during acute disease. Ileus precludes oral antibiotics from reaching the area of inflammation and necrosis. Therefore prophylactic antibiotics for intestinal microflora hold little hope for the prevention of NEC.

Nearly 90% of all cases of NEC are best described as a form of inflammatory bowel disease related in some manner to feeding. Figure 9.1 illustrates the multifactorial relationship of feeding associated NEC. The preterm infant is in precarious balance. Mucosal defences, intestinal motility and the gut microcirculation have a limited ability to withstand an insult, luminal or vascular in origin, and recover fully. Aggressive feedings provide undigested substrate for microflora. An altered intestinal flora fermentation rate, adherence or translocation can readily overwhelm this fragile ecosystem.

Counterproductive and potentially dangerous therapeutic approaches target intestinal mast cells, neutrophils and intestinal circulation. Mast cell stabilizers are effective in pulmonary disease but are not beneficial in the intestine. Mucosal mast cells are of a different phenotype, and no therapeutic agent in this class is available for an intestinal site of action. Specific neutrophil antagonists which may help to limit the extension of tissue injury in NEC cannot be

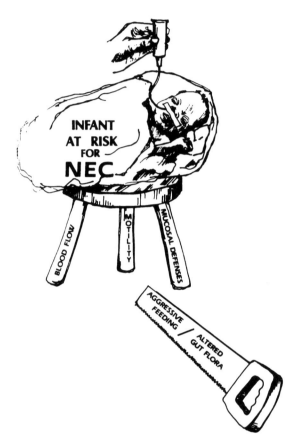

Figure 9.1 Intestinal blood flow, motility and mucosal defences, three factors which protect the preterm infant from NEC may be overwhelmed by aggressive feeding or altered intestinal flora.

used in newborns because of the high risk for sepsis. Selective vaso-dilators for intestinal circulation are not available. Systemic vasodilators could result in systemic hypotension and decreased mesenteric perfusion.

Table 9.6 summarizes therapeutic approaches that may be useful in preterm infants to prevent NEC or lessen its severity. The iatrogenic component of neonatal inflammatory bowel disease (NEC) is exces-sive feeding in the face of unrecognized intestinal dysfunction. A use-ful practice for modifying this form of disease is to feed small volumes within the first several days after birth[25]. This 'gut priming' minimizes intestinal mucosal atrophy and allows for a more functional intestine

Table 9.6 Prevention of necrotizing enterocolitis

* Modify feeding practices
  Low volume – 'gut priming' during acute illness
  Cautious incremental volumes
* Better formulae for preterm infants
  Improved digestibility/absorption
  Addition of 'breast milk' factors
    Lactoferrin
    Immunoglobulins
    Prostaglandins
* Enhancement of mucosal barrier
  Antenatal steroids
  Growth factors (epidermal, insulin-like)
  Prostaglandin E analogues
* Improve motility
* Early detection of intestinal dysfunction
* Inflammatory mediator antagonists
* Free radical scavengers
  Superoxide dismutase
* L-Arginine

and a successful progression of feedings after the acute illness has resolved. Feedings should be monitored with stooling frequency. Failure to stool in the face of advancing feedings suggests a potential motility disorder and establishes conditions favourable for bacterial growth and intestinal injury.

Feedings provide substrate to the intestinal microflora, a significant concern because intestinal function decreases with increasing prematurity. Although there is no ideal formula for the preterm infant, improved formulae may minimize the impact of malabsorption. The addition of breast milk factors to formulae may promote mucosal growth as well as modify intestinal colonization[25]. Lactoferrin and immunoglobulins may select for desirable intestinal microflora. Prostaglandins and immunoglobulins may enhance barrier function[42,43].

Antenatal steroids have decreased the incidence of necrotizing enterocolitis as well as surfactant deficiency syndrome. This is presumed to be due to the enhancement of the mucosal barrier. Epidermal and insulin-like growth factors promote a more luxurious villus formation. Prostaglandin E analogues (e.g. misoprostol) have been shown to enhance the mucosal barrier and promote microvillus development[42]. Prostaglandin E analogues also stimulate intestinal motility, which, although undesirable in adult inflammatory bowel disease, may be helpful for the preterm infant.

Intestinal motility is a function of the maturity of the enteric nervous system[24]. Variability in maturity may occur, even in infants of the same gestational age. Pharmaceuticals that accelerate the maturity of the enteric nervous system would be most effective. Prokinetic agents, cisapride and erythromycin, have not been studied in a randomized, controlled fashion in preterm infants. Since they function to integrate a poorly coordinated but mature enteric nervous system, they may not be effective in the smallest infants at greatest risk. Gastric residuals, often used as a harbinger of NEC, only indicate delayed gastric emptying and are a poor marker of distal intestinal dysfunction. The volume of the residual may vary according to catheter tip position. Delayed gastric emptying may be a late sign of significant ileocolonic disease, suggesting a generalized intestinal ileus. One proven marker is the gastrocolic reflex, the infant's capacity to stool in response to increased feedings. Delayed stooling has been shown to precede NEC by 3–5 days[44].

Biochemical markers may detect intestinal inflammation before the onset of any clinical symptomatology. Positive stool reducing substances, breath hydrogen and urinary D-lactate all indicate carbohydrate malabsorption but are poor predictors of intestinal damage. Biochemical markers of inflammation, such as urinary histamine for mast cell activation, myeloperoxidase (neutrophil activation) and leukotrienes, may prove to be an early warning system for a reactive intestine at risk and ill prepared for an aggressive dietary challenge.

Drug antagonists for specific inflammatory mediators are a potential but yet unproven therapeutic approach. Since inflammation is a complex process and involves numerous components which are necessary for homeostasis, agents that may be effective in animal models in short term experiments may not prove to be effective in preterm infants. Platelet activating factor and TNF-α are released after the initiation of intestinal injury. While both remain intriguing mediators, it is unlikely that drugs antagonizing these agents will be available for adult diseases in the near future, let alone for high risk neonates. By the time NEC is evident, many mediators have already played their role. The best 'theoretical' intervention would be prophylaxis because the precise timing of injury in the clinical setting is unknown.

Two potentially useful therapeutic pharmaceuticals are superoxide dismutase and L-arginine. A human recombinant superoxide dismutase is available and has been used in humans following transplantation to scavenge free radicals. Its safety is proven and it may be potentially effective in limiting the propagation of incipient inflammatory bowel disease[40]. However, prophylactic use of superoxide dismutase would be prohibitively expensive.

Nitric oxide release is exaggerated in models of NEC and interventions aimed at nitric oxide synthase have been proven to be beneficial in other forms of inflammatory bowel disease. Supplemental L-arginine attenuates the intestinal inflammation in the acid–casein model of NEC in piglets[45] and in platelet activating factor induced intestinal necrosis in rats[46]. However, nitric oxide may prevent or promote gut injury[47], depending on the enzyme source, amounts produced and interactions with other oxidants[48]. Thus, while nitric oxide may be an attractive therapeutic target, considerable experimentation is necessary before clinical intervention is possible.

In summary, ischaemia–reperfusion injury and specific enteropathogenic organisms are less essential than previously postulated. The intestinal dysfunction, malabsorption and poor motility of fed preterm infants precipitates intestinal inflammation. Recognition of inflammatory bowel disease as the dominant form of NEC allows for a broad range of scientific approaches to decrease its incidence and severity.

REFERENCES

1. Kliegman RM, Walker WA and Yolken RH. Necrotizing enterocolitis: research agenda for a disease of unknown etiology and pathogenesis. *Pediatr Res* 1993;**34:**701–708.
2. Stoll BJ. Epidemiology of necrotizing enterocolitis. *Clin Perinatol* 1994;**21:**205–218.
3. Uauy RD, Fanaroff AA, Korones SB, Phillips EA, Philips JB and Wright LL. Necrotizing enterocolitis in very low birth weight infants: biodemographic and clinical correlates. *J Pediatr* 1991;**119:**630–638.
4. deGamarra E, Helardot P, Moriette G, Murat I and Relier JP. Necrotizing enterocolitis in full-term newborns. *Biol Neonate* 1983;**44:**185–192.
5. Thilo EH, Lezarte RA and Hernandez JA. Necrotizing enterocolitis in the first 24 hours of life. *Pediatrics* 1984;**73:**476–480.
6. Andrews DA, Sawin RS, Ledbetter DE, Schaller RT and Hatch EI. Necrotizing enterocolitis in term infants. *Am J Surg* 1990;**159:**507–509.
7. Stoll BJ, Kanto WP, Glass RI, Nahmias AJ and Brann AW. Epidemiology of necrotizing enterocolitis: a case control study. *J Pediatr* 1980;**96:**447–452.
8. Kanto WP, Wilson R, Breart GL, Zierler S, Purohit DM and Peckham GJ. Perinatal events and necrotizing enterocolitis in premature infants. *Am J Dis Child* 1987;**141:**167–169.

9. Marchildon MB, Buck BE and Abdenour G. Necrotizing enterocolitis in the unfed infant. *J Pediatr Surg* 1982;**17**:620–624.

10. Samm M, Curtis-Cohen M, Keller M and Chawla H. Necrotizing enterocolitis in infants of multiple gestation. *Am J Dis Child* 1986;**140**:937–939.

11. Clark DA, Barkemeyer BM and Miller MJS. Perinatal hypoxic-ischemic risk factors and necrotizing enterocolitis. *Pediatr Res* 1993;**32**:207.

12. Ryder RW, Shelton JD and Guinan ME. Necrotizing enterocolitis: a prospective multicenter investigation. *Am J Epidemiol* 1980;**112**:113–123.

13. Wilson R, Kanto WP Jr, McCarthy BJ and Feldman RA. Age at onset of necrotizing enterocolitis: risk factors in small infants. *Am J Dis Child* 1982;**136**:814–816.

14. Dénes J, Gergely K, Wohlmuth G and Leb J. Necrotizing enterocolitis of premature infants. *Surgery* 1970;**68**:558–561.

15. Wiswell TE, Robertson CF, Jones TA and Tuttle DJ. Necrotizing enterocolitis in full-term infants: a case control study. *Am J Dis Child* 1988;**142**:532–535.

16. Covert RF, Neu J, Elliott MJ, Rea JL and Gimotty PA. Factors associated with age of onset of necrotizing enterocolitis. *Am J Perinatol* 1989;**6**:455–460.

17. Clark DA, Thompson JE, Weiner LB and McMillan JA. Necrotizing enterocolitis: intraluminal biochemistry in human neonates and a rabbit model. *Pediatr Res* 1985;**19**:919–921.

18. Goldman HI. Feeding and necrotizing enterocolitis. *Am J Dis Child* 1980;**134**:553–555.

19. Clark DA and Miller MJS. Intraluminal pathogenesis of necrotizing enterocolitis. *J Pediatr* 1990;**117**:S64–67.

20. Willoughby RE and Pickering LK. Necrotizing enterocolitis and infection. *Clin Perinatol* 1994;**21**:307–316.

21. Rotbart HA and Levin MJ. How contagious is necrotizing enterocolitis? *Pediatr Infect Dis J* 1983;**2**:406–410.

22. Carbonaro CA, Clark DA and Elseviers D. A bacterial pathogenicity determinant associated with necrotizing enterocolitis. *Microb Pathol* 1988;**5**:427–436.

23. Gupta S, Morris JG, Panigrahi P, Nataro JP, Glass RI and Gewolb IH. Endemic necrotizing enterocolitis: lack of association with a specific infectious agent. *Pediatr Infect Dis J* 1994;**13**:728–734.

24. Berseth C. Gut motility and the pathogenesis of necrotizing enterocolitis. *Clin Perinatol* 1994;**21**:263–270.

25. Miller MJS, Sadowska-Krowicka H, Jeng AY et al. Substance P levels in experimental ileitis in the guinea pig: effects of misoprostol. *Am J Physiol* 1993;**265**:G321–330.

26. LaGamma EF and Browne LE. Feeding practices for infants weighing less than 1500 g at birth and the pathogenesis of necrotizing enterocolitis. *Clin Perinatol* 1994;**21**:271–306.

27. Stevenson DK, Shahin SM, Ostrander CR et al. Breath hydrogen in

preterm infants: correlation with changes in bacterial colonization of the gastrointestinal tract. *J Pediatr* 1982;**101**:607–610.

28. Garcia J, Smith FR and Cucinell SA. Urinary D-lactate excretion in infants with necrotizing enterocolitis. *J Pediatr* 1984;**104**:268–270.

29. Miller MJS, Witherly SA and Clark DA. Casein: a milk protein with diverse biological consequences. *Proc Soc Exp Biol Med* 1990;**195**:143–159.

30. Miller MJS, Zhang X-J, Gu X, Tenore E and Clark DA. Exaggerated intestinal histamine release by casein and casein hydrolysate but not whey hydrolysate. *Scand J Gastroenterol* 1991;**26**:379–384.

31. Crissinger KD. Regulation of hemodynamics and oxygenation in developing intestine: insight into the pathogenesis of necrotizing enterocolitis. *Acta Paediatr Suppl* 1994;**396**:8–10.

32. Buescher ES. Host defense mechanisms of human milk. *Clin Perinatol* 1994;**21**:247–262.

33. Nowicki PT and Nankervis CA. The role of the circulation in the pathogenesis of necrotizing enterocolitis. *Clin Perinatol* 1994;**211**:219–234.

34. Scheifele DW. Role of bacterial toxins in neonatal necrotizing enterocolitis. *J Pediatr* 1990;S44–47.

35. Miller MJS and Clark DA. Profile and sites of eicosanoid release in experimental necrotizing enterocolitis. *Adv Prostaglandin Thromboxane Leukotriene Res* 1989;**19**:556–559.

36. Morecroft JA, Spitz L, Hamilton PA and Holmes SJ. Plasma cytokine levels in necrotizing enterocolitis. *Acta Paediatr Suppl* 1994;**396**:18–20.

37. Clark DA, Fornabaio DM, McNeill H, Mulane KM and Miller MJS. Contribution of oxygen-derived free radicals to experimental necrotizing enterocolitis. *Am J Pathol* 1988;**130**:537–542.

38. Caplan MS and MacKendrick W. Inflammatory mediators and intestinal injury. *Clin Perinatol* 1994;**21**:235–246.

39. Miller MJS, Zhang X-J, Sadowska-Krowicka H et al. Nitric oxide release in response to gut injury. *Scand J Gastroenterol* 1993;**28**:149–154.

40. Miller MJS, McNeill H, Mullane KM, Caravella SJ and Clark DA. SOD prevents damage and attenuates eicosanoid release in a rabbit model of necrotizing enterocolitis. *Am J Physiol* 1988;**255**:G556–565.

41. Vasan U and Gotoff SP. Prevention of neonatal necrotizing enterocolitis. *Clin Perinatol* 1994;**21**:425–436.

42. Miller MJS, Zhang X-J, Gu X and Clark DA. Acute intestinal injury induced by organic acids and casein: prevention by intraluminal misoprostol. *Gastroenterology* 1991;**101**:22–30.

43. Eibl MM, Wolf WM and Furnkranz H. Prevention of necrotizing enterocolitis in low birth weight infants by IgA-IgG feeding. *N Engl J Med* 1988;**319**:1–5.

44. Wright LL, Uauy RD, Younes N, Fanaroff AA, Korones SB and Philips JB. Rapid advances in feeding increase the risk of necrotizing enterocolitis in very low birth weight infants. *Pediatr Res* 1993;**33**:313 (abstract).

45. DiLorenzo M, Bass J and Krantis A. Use of L-arginine in the treatment of experimental necrotizing enterocolitis. *J Pediatr Surg* 1995;**30**:235–241.

46. MacKendrick W, Caplan M and Hsueh W. Endogenous nitric oxide protects against platelet activating factor-induced bowel injury in the rat. *Pediatr Res* 1993;**34**:222–228.
47. Miller MJS, Sadowska-Krowicka H, Chotinaruemol S, Kakkis JL and Clark DA. Amelioration of chronic ileitis by nitric oxide synthase inhibition. *J Pharmacol Exp Ther* 1994;**264**:11–16.
48. Miller MSJ and Ribbons KA. Nitric oxide and inflammatory bowel disease; opportunities for a new approach. *Prog Inflamm Bowel Dis* 1994;**15**:9–15.

10

Gene Therapy for the Lung

Barbara Warner and Jonathan Wispè

INTRODUCTION

In this chapter we shall discuss human gene therapy as it pertains to the lung. The field of gene therapy is evolving at a rapid rate, therefore our objective is not to detail specifically the current human trials, because this information would be rapidly dated; rather, we hope to demonstrate the exciting possibilities of gene therapy, and stress the difficulties and potential risks. We shall briefly review the molecular biology of genes. Next we shall describe the currently available methods of gene transfer, emphasizing the advantages and disadvantages of each. Finally, we shall review lung diseases, which are candidates for gene therapy.

The lung is an ideal candidate organ for gene therapy. It is afflicted by inherited diseases, cancers and inflammatory processes that could be amenable to gene therapy. In addition, the lung has a large surface area which is accessible to direct administration of 'therapeutic' genes. Because of these factors and the significance, medically and economically, of pulmonary diseases, the lung has been a natural area of emphasis of research for gene therapies.

BACKGROUND MOLECULAR AND CELLULAR BIOLOGY

In order to understand the methodology and prospective uses of gene therapy, it is important to understand the components involved: DNA, genes, proteins and cells.

Eukaryotic Gene Transcription

DNA is composed of four nucleotide bases: adenine (A), guanine (G), cytosine (C) and thymidine (T). A *gene* is defined as a region of DNA that encodes a functional protein or ribonucleic acid. The region on the chromosome which encompasses a gene (Figure 10.1) includes: *exons*, which code for the amino acid sequence contained in a protein; *introns*, which are intervening DNA sequences that do not encode information used to assemble the protein; and *promoters and enhancers*, which are non-coding sequences of DNA that regulate gene expression. Promoters and enhancers determine when the gene is expressed, confer tissue specificity and determine the level of expression.

The information contained in DNA is transcribed into RNA, which is translated into protein (Figure 10.1). Messenger RNA (mRNA) carries the information in the exons of genes using a three letter genetic alphabet. This alphabet consists of groups of three nucleotides, called codons. Each codon specifies a single amino acid. A mutation occurs when nucleotides are deleted, inserted or changed from the normal sequence. Changes in the nucleotides alter the codons and ultimately the amino acid sequence of the protein. Alterations in the amino acid sequence result in changes in protein structure and function, which are the bases of many genetic diseases.

The mRNA molecules leave the nucleus and direct synthesis of protein on cytoplasmic ribosomes. In the laboratory, cytoplasmic mRNA is often copied back into DNA. These artificial DNA molecules contain all the information originally present in the RNA, and are more stable and easily manipulated. These molecules are called

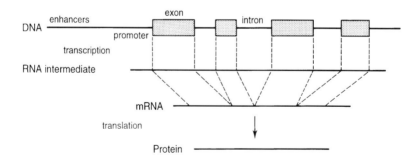

Figure 10.1 Structure of eukaryotic genes.

complementary DNAs (cDNAs), and are the molecules actually used for gene therapy.

For gene transfer to occur, two components are required: the DNA to be transferred, and the vehicle used to transfer it. The DNA to be transferred is usually not the full length gene. Complete genes, with both introns and exons, are usually too large to incorporate into the available transfer vehicles. Typically cDNAs which include only the information needed for a functional protein are used in gene transfer. The DNA sequences that confer control of endogenous gene expression are usually omitted.

Gene Transfer

Transfer of foreign DNA into host cells is a multistep process. The DNA must be internalized by the cell, released into the cytoplasm and transferred to the nucleus. In the gene transfer systems to be discussed, internalization occurs by endocytosis. Endocytosis is the process by which the plasma membrane invaginates around a particle until it is surrounded and contained within a new intracellular membrane. In receptor mediated endocytosis a specific macromolecule (ligand), which binds to a cell receptor, is attached to the DNA to be transferred. After binding, the receptor–ligand–DNA complex undergoes endocytosis and internalization. The endocytic vesicle is mildly acidified, then fuses with a lysosome. Lysosomes contain proteases and other hydrolytic enzymes that degrade the contents of the endosome. For DNA to reach the nucleus intact, it must be released from the endosome before exposure to lysosomal proteases and nucleases. After release into the cytoplasm, the DNA is transferred to the nucleus, where it may remain separate from the host cell chromosomes (episomal) or insert into the host genome (integrate).

Episomal DNA is transcribed independently of the host cell DNA. Cell division results in transfer of the episomal DNA to only one daughter cell. A series of cell divisions will have a significant dilutional effect on the transferred DNA. Because of this 'dilution', episomal DNA will not provide long lasting expression. For treatment of inherited genetic diseases, episomal DNA will require repeated administration. For acquired diseases, episomal DNA could provide expression during the course of a limited illness. DNA which integrates into the host DNA is transcribed with the host DNA. With cell division, a copy of the integrated DNA is passed on to each daughter cell. For correction of genetic diseases, integrated therapeutic DNA could potentially induce a permanent correction. Because the transferred DNA inserts randomly into the host genome, there is a risk of inserting into and disrupting important endogenous genes. Insertion could also activate an oncogene or cause aberrant cellular growth and development of a malignancy. This process is called *insertional mutagenesis* and is one of the most worrisome aspects of gene therapy.

GENE TRANSFER SYSTEMS

The process of introducing DNA into cells is called transfection. There are two general techniques for transfection of eukaryotic cells: physical or chemical methods, and biological viral vectors. Physical/chemical techniques include calcium phosphate precipitation, electroporation, microinjection, liposomes and DNA–protein conjugates. Although the others are used in the laboratory, only liposomes and DNA–protein conjugates appear practical for clinical use. Viral vectors used for gene transfer to the lung include adenovirus (Ad), adeno associated virus (AAV) and retrovirus.

Physical Methods of Gene Transfer

Liposomes
Lipofection is a process in which lipid vesicles (liposomes) are used to introduce DNA into cells. Liposomes are spherical bilayers of phospholipids, with aqueous interiors that can entrap soluble molecules, like DNA. Liposomes enter a cell by endocytosis, eventually fusing with a lysosome. Several problems have limited the efficiency of liposome mediated gene transfer: the entrapment efficiency of DNA into liposomes is low; intravenously administered liposomes are rapidly cleared by the reticuloendothelial system, which may prevent them from reaching the target organ; and lysosomal degradation of the incorporated DNA is high. The efficiency of liposome mediated gene transfer is increased by including positively charged (cationic) lipids in the liposome. Cationic lipid binds negatively charged DNA, increasing the amount of DNA associated with the liposome. The net charge of the DNA–liposome complex is positive, which enhances the interaction with the negatively charged cell surface and increases cellular uptake. There also appears to be less lysosomal degradation of the DNA in cationic lysosomes[1,2]. Various mixtures of cationic lipids have been used for lipofection. Lipofectin[3] (marketed as Lipofectin™ Reagent, GIBCO BRL, Gaithersburg, MD), uses equal

parts of the cationic lipid N-[1-(2,3-dioleoyloxy)propyl]-N,N,N-trimethylammonium chloride (DOTMA) and the neutral lipid dioleoylphosphatidylcholine (DOPE). Lipofectin has been used to introduce DNA into animal lung by intratracheal instillation[4], by tracheal aerosolization[5] or by intravenous injection[6–8]. Cationic liposomes have been used to transfer the cystic fibrosis transmembrane regulator (CFTR) gene to the respiratory epithelium of mice and nasal epithelium of humans. Hyde et al[9] demonstrated transfer of the CFTR gene and functional correction of chloride ion transport in transgenic cystic fibrosis (CF) mice using cationic liposomes. Zhu et al[6] reported CFTR expression in lungs, lymph nodes, bone marrow and spleen for up to 9 weeks following a single intravenous injection of DOTMA/DOPA/CFTR DNA in mice. Most recently, Caplen et al[10] used cationic liposomes to transfer the CFTR gene to the nasal epithelium of nine patients with cystic fibrosis.

Tissue specificity can be improved by adding tissue specific antibodies or antigens to the surface of liposomes which are directed against antigens or receptors on the target cell. Hughes et al[11] constructed liposomes containing an antibody directed against an endothelial cell protein that is expressed almost exclusively in the lung. When these liposomes were ^{125}I-labelled and injected intravenously or intraperitoneally into mice, accumulation was 22 times higher in lung than any other tissue. An alternative means of achieving lung specific expression is the inclusion of lung specific DNA promoter elements in the transferred gene. Promoter elements from the lung surfactant protein-C (SP-C) gene direct gene expression specifically to type II respiratory epithelial cells[12]. Hazinski et al[13] linked the SP-C gene promoter to a marker gene, β-galactosidase. This DNA complex was incorporated into liposomes and administered intratracheally into rats. Staining for β-galactosidase was seen only in type II respiratory epithelial cells, consistent with the cell specific expression of SP-C.

DNA delivered by liposomes and immunoliposomes remains susceptible to lysosomal degradation. To prevent this, the composition of some liposomes has been altered so that at the mildly acidic pH of the newly internalized endosome (pH 5.0–6.5), the liposome fuses with and destabilizes the endocytic membrane, causing it to release contained DNA into the cell. These pH sensitive liposomes are constructed by including phosphatidylethanolamine (PE) into the liposome. At acidic pHs, PE causes the liposome to fuse with the endosome membrane and release the DNA into the cytoplasm before lysosomal degradation[14].

DNA-protein conjugates

Polymers of positively charged amino acids, such as lysine, have also been used to transfer DNA. The positively charged polylysine will bind the negatively charged DNA. The protein–DNA complex is taken up into the cell by endocytosis. Tissue specific delivery is increased by linking ligands for cell surface receptors to the protein–DNA complex. The polylysine–DNA–ligand complex binds to specific cell surface receptors, and enters the cell by receptor mediated endocytosis. In vitro, DNA has been transferred to cultured respiratory epithelial cells by linking surfactant protein-A (SP-A), a lung specific protein, to a polylysine–DNA complex[15]. In vivo, DNA transfer was accomplished by linking the polymeric immunoglobulin receptor (pIgR) to the polylysine. Intravenous administration of a DNA–polylysine–pIgR complex to rats resulted in expression of transferred DNA in lung and liver[16].

The polylysine complexes are internalized as endosomes, which means that the DNA is susceptible to lysosomal degradation. To limit degradation, viral capsid proteins that destabilize endosomal membranes have been included with the protein–DNA complexes. Following receptor mediated endocytosis, the endosomes are acidified, which causes a conformational change of capsid proteins. This conformational change disrupts the endosomal membrane, and the endosomal contents are released into the cytoplasm. Proteins from both influenza virus[17] and adenovirus[18,19] have been used to increase the DNA delivery to the cytoplasm before lysosomal degradation.

Use of lipofection and DNA–protein conjugates has advantages over biological viral methods of DNA transfer: (1) they can deliver large DNA fragments; (2) there is no viral genetic material present; (3) minimal toxicities have been reported; (4) DNA can be transferred to both dividing and non-dividing cells; and (5) the physical/chemical vectors are easily manufactured. With physical DNA transfer, the DNA remains episomal, alleviating the concern about insertional mutagenesis. However, cell division will 'dilute' the transferred DNA and limit expression. Use of physical DNA methods for inherited diseases may therefore be limited because of the need for repeated dosing. Most importantly, DNA transfer with either liposomes or protein complexes is still inefficient. Duration and level of expression varies greatly, as does cellular specificity of gene transfer. Before these technologies become practical for human gene therapy, improvements will need to be made to improve cellular uptake, decrease lysosomal degradation and improve organ specific targeting.

Biological Viral Vectors

Adenoviral vectors

Adenoviruses (Ads) are a common cause of respiratory infections in humans. They are double stranded DNA viruses that replicate within the host cell nucleus. Respiratory epithelial cells have a membrane receptor which specifically binds adenoviral coat proteins. After binding to the cell surface, the Ad enters the cell by receptor mediated endocytosis and forms an endosome which contains the viral particle. The endosome is mildly acidified, which induces a conformational change in the adenoviral capsid and causes endosomal rupture. The contents of the endosome are released into the cytoplasm before lysosomal fusion and degradation. Once in the cytoplasm the uncoated viral DNA migrates to the nucleus where it remains extrachromosomal. This endosomalytic property of the adenoviral proteins increases the efficiency of DNA transfer. The Ad used for gene transfer is not capable of replication. These 'replication deficient' viral vectors are made by removal of the region of DNA that is required to initiate viral transcription, the E1 region (Figure 10.2). Deletion of the E1 and often the E3 regions provides space for insertion of the foreign gene. To prepare the recombinant adenoviral DNA, which contains the foreign DNA for transfer, it is transfected into a packaging cell which puts an adenoviral coat around it. The recombinant adenovirus is capable of infecting cells and directing transcription of the newly inserted foreign DNA, but is not capable of replicating adenoviral DNA[20]. Adenoviral vectors have been used for the transfer of numerous genes to a variety of target organs. They have been used for transfer of the CFTR and α_1 antitrypsin (α_1-AT) cDNAs to the respiratory epithelium in several animals[21–26], and are presently being used in phase I trials of CFTR transfer to the nasal and respiratory epithelium of humans with cystic fibrosis[27–30].

The advantages of using adenoviral vectors for human gene therapy

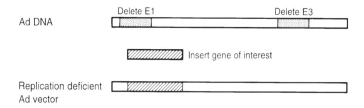

Figure 10.2 Construction of Ad vectors for gene transfer.

to the lung include the presence of Ad receptors on respiratory epithelial cells, the high efficiency of gene transfer, the ability to infect non-replicating cells and the lack of viral associated malignancies. There are several disadvantages to Ad based gene therapy. The transferred DNA does not integrate into the host cell DNA. Cell division leads to dilution of the transferred gene and limits gene expression. Treatment of inherited diseases with adenoviral vectors will require repeated administration. More importantly, adenoviral administration elicits a vigorous immune response. An early acute cytopathic neutrophil phase, which peaks at 48 hours, is followed by a cytotoxic T cell mediated phase, which resolves by 3–4 weeks. This inflammatory response will limit the duration and efficiency of gene expression, and may cause lung injury[31–34]. It now appears that small amounts of adenoviral protein are made, despite the E1 deletion, which elicit the immune response. Investigators are now attempting to minimize the immune response by further modifying the adenoviral DNA[23].

Conjugated adenovirus–protein–DNA complexes
Replication deficient Ad has also been used in combination with DNA–polylysine complexes for gene transfer. The DNA to be transferred is complexed to the polylysine. The adenoviral particles are used for their endosomalytic capabilities and are replication deficient, but contain no foreign DNA. The DNA–polylysine complexes are mixed with the adenoviral particles and co-administered to cells. Both the DNA–polylysine complexes and the adenoviral particles enter the cell through endocytosis. Some of the internalized endosomes will contain both adenoviral particles and DNA–protein complexes. After internalization and endosomal acidification, conformational changes in the adenoviral proteins cause rupture of the endosome and release of the co-internalized DNA–polylysine complexes into the cytoplasm[19,35]. Delivery of DNA can be further enhanced by attaching the Ad particle to the DNA–protein complexes chemically[36,37], or with antibodies[38,39]. With Ad–DNA–protein complexes, smaller amounts of Ad are administered, which should decrease the inflammatory response and increase the efficiency of the DNA–protein complexes. Ad–DNA–protein complexes have been used for gene transfer to the respiratory epithelium of rats[40] and for the transfer of α_1 antitrypsin to hepatocytes[41].

Adeno associated virus
Adeno associated virus (AAV) is a small, replication deficient, human parvovirus that requires co-infection with Ad or herpesvirus

to replicate. When cells are infected with AAV, the viral DNA stably integrates into the host cell genome. AAV based vectors are promising for gene therapy because they efficiently infect the respiratory epithelium, do not require rapidly dividing cells and are not known to cause carcinogenesis in humans[42]. Wild type AAV preferentially inserts into the human genome at a specific site on chromosome 19. Theoretically, this should decrease the risk of insertional mutagenesis. Current AAV vectors, however, have not retained this property, and there is evidence that, in vivo, AAV remains episomal. There are also technical problems with AAV vectors. The small size of AAV (4.68 kb) limits the size of foreign DNA that can be incorporated to about 4.5 kb, and it has not been possible to produce AAV in high titres. However, AAV has been used to transfer the CFTR gene to cultured respiratory epithelial cells[43] and to rabbit lung in vivo[44].

Retroviruses

Retroviruses are RNA viruses that form a double stranded DNA intermediate after infecting host cells. The double stranded viral DNA then randomly integrates into the host genome. Stable integration into the host genome will maintain gene expression through subsequent cell division, but also carries the risk of disrupting normal genes and of insertional mutagenesis[45]. Retroviral integration and gene transfer require rapidly dividing cells[46]. Respiratory epithelial cells normally divide slowly, making retroviruses a poor candidate for gene therapy of the lung. Retroviruses are used most commonly in the treatment of cancers and have been successfully used in the treatment of various lung cancers[47,48].

CANDIDATE DISEASES

Candidate diseases for gene therapy fall into three broad categories: (1) classic genetic diseases, which follow a mendelian pattern of inheritance; (2) complex genetic diseases, which are often multifactorial in their aetiologies; and (3) acquired diseases[49]. Each of these categories requires different approaches for genetic therapies. Classic genetic diseases that result in a deficiency of an important protein will require lifelong replacement therapy and best results may be achieved by cell or organ specific replacement. In contrast, therapeutic objectives for acquired diseases may be directed towards correcting a temporary condition or preventing complications of the disease.

Classic Genetic Diseases

These are diseases that are caused by a single gene defect. There are several requirements for a genetic disease to be eligible for gene therapy. The sequence and structure of the disease gene must be known, the functional properties of the gene product must be determined and, finally, the target cells or organ must be identified. The presence of a single gene defect does not make gene therapy straightforward. Genetic diseases are often complex multiorgan diseases, which makes identification of a target organ difficult. They also require lifelong treatment. Three genetic diseases of the lung have been evaluated for treatment by gene therapy: cystic fibrosis, α_1-AT deficiency, and hereditary surfactant protein B (SP-B) deficiency. Of these, only gene therapy for treatment of cystic fibrosis has advanced to clinical trials.

Cystic fibrosis

Cystic fibrosis is the most common lethal autosomal recessive disorder in Caucasians. The genetic defect has been characterized[50]. The affected gene, the cystic fibrosis transmembrane conductance regulator (CFTR), encodes for a 1480 amino acid protein which functions as a chloride channel. Lung disease is the major source of morbidity and mortality in cystic fibrosis and gene therapy has been aimed at introducing the CFTR cDNA into respiratory epithelial cells. Various gene transfer methods are being tried. Adenoviral vectors[27–30] and cationic liposomes[10,51] are being used in phase I clinical trials. These initial trials are primarily aimed at evaluating the safety of these vectors in patients with cystic fibrosis, particularly since Ad vectors have been shown to elicit an immune response in various animal models (see above). AAV has been used to transfer CFTR to respiratory epithelial cells in vitro[43] and to rabbit lung in vivo[44]. In rabbits, AAV-CFTR was introduced intrabronchially and both CFTR transcripts and CFTR protein were detected for 6 months after administration, without obvious toxicity. A major hurdle in the use of AAV-CFTR is the inability to produce the high concentrations of virus needed to treat humans. Despite these problems, the initial results are promising and human trials with AAV-CFTR are under consideration. Retroviral vectors have been used for the successful transfer of CFTR and other genes to the respiratory epithelium in vitro[52,53]. The low turnover rate of the respiratory epithelium remains a major problem for human retroviral based gene therapy.

α₁-Antitrypsin deficiency

The antiprotease, α_1-AT, is produced by the liver and protects the lung from destruction by neutrophil elastase, a powerful proteolytic enzyme. In hereditary α_1-AT deficiency, mutations in the α_1-AT gene result in a deficiency of circulating levels of α_1-AT. Unopposed proteolytic activity results in destruction of alveolar architecture and causes progressive pulmonary emphysema. Human gene therapy for α_1-AT deficiency has targeted replacement genes to hepatocytes[54,55], endothelial cells[56] and respiratory epithelial cells[21,57,58]. The most promising results have been obtained using adenoviral vectors to transfer genetic material to liver or lung. Kay[41] demonstrated that injection of an Ad vector containing the human α_1-AT cDNA into the portal vein of mice resulted in protective levels of α_1-antitrypsin. Rosenfeld and colleagues[21] intratracheally administered Ad–human α_1-AT to rats, and detected human α_1-AT in the epithelial lining for at least 1 week after treatment. The human α_1-AT cDNA has also been transferred to the lungs of rabbits using cationic liposomes injected intravenously or aerosolized intratracheally. Both methods of administration resulted in expression of the human α_1-AT in the lung for at least 7 days without notable toxicity.

Surfactant protein-B deficiency

Hereditary SP-B deficiency is a lethal pulmonary disorder of newborns that presents with a clinical and histological picture of congenital alveolar proteinosis[59]. Fullterm newborns present with intractable respiratory failure which is resistant to surfactant replacement and maximal medical management. SP-B deficiency has been uniformly fatal. Histologically, alveoli are filled with lipid and protein rich material. Alveolar material from these patients is deficient in SP-B and a mutation in the SP-B gene has recently been demonstrated in multiple kindreds of patients presenting with congenital alveolar proteinosis[60]. Yei et al[61] used an adenoviral vector to transfer the human SP-B cDNA to respiratory epithelial cells in vitro and in vivo. Cotton rats, intratracheally administered Ad containing the human SP-B cDNA, produced levels of human SP-B within 48 hours of treatment. At the same time a dose dependent inflammatory response characteristic of Ad vectors was evident in Ad–SP-B treated animals. These findings support the concept that gene therapy can provide a potentially life saving new mode of therapy for infants, but also demonstrate the problems with currently available delivery systems.

Complex Genetic Diseases

The aetiology of diseases such as cancer and cardiovascular disease is multifactorial, with environmental and genetic components involved in their pathogenesis. Gene therapy for these diseases can be directed towards augmenting normal cellular functions, or towards providing a new therapeutic function.

Lung cancer is one model of how gene therapy is being applied to complex genetic diseases. Gene therapy for cancer is usually done ex vivo. Cells from the tumour are surgically removed, transfected with the new DNA in the laboratory, then reinserted into the animal or patient. Retrovirus vectors are commonly used for gene transfer in tumour cells because they efficiently transfer DNA in rapidly dividing cells. Three different strategies for gene therapy of cancer have been considered. Transferred genes can (1) augment the normal immune response, (2) kill tumour cells, or (3) suppress tumour formation. The normal immune response may be augmented by adding the genes of cytokines which are toxic to tumour cells, such as tumour necrosis factor[62]. Alternatively, the cancer cell can be made to express a foreign HLA antigen to which the host immune system will react[63]. One of the most common genes which kills tumour cells is the herpes simplex thymidine kinase gene (HSVTK). Thymidine kinase converts a non-toxic prodrug, gancyclovir, to a cytotoxic phosphorylated form. Cancer therapy with the TK cDNA requires that it be expressed only in tumour cells. To direct in vivo therapy, tissue specific promoters can be included with the HSVTK cDNA. Lung specific expression of TK was accomplished by including a promoter from the human SP-A gene in a retroviral vector with TK[48]. This approach limited gancyclovir cytotoxicity to lung cells. Finally, mutations in the tumour suppresser gene p53 are common in human lung cancer. Lack of a functional p53 protein disrupts control of cell proliferation and facilitates oncogenesis. Because the normal p53 gene product is dominant over the non-functional mutant, insertion of a normal p53 cDNA into a cancer cell can establish regulated cell division. Treatment of lung tumour cells which contained a p53 mutation, with a retroviral vector containing the wild type p53, significantly inhibited tumour growth both in cell culture and in a mouse model[64].

Acquired Diseases

As the molecular basis of many acquired diseases is better understood, the potential for gene therapy will increase. For many acquired diseases, expression of the transferred gene would ideally be limited to the period necessary to treat the disease. For this reason episomal vectors are more appropriate for treatment of acquired diseases. Lung injury occurs with systemic sepsis, the adult respiratory distress syndrome (ARDS), oxygen toxicity, and use of radiation and chemotherapy in treatment of cancer. Gene transfer techniques to prevent or treat these forms of acute lung injury have been limited to the laboratory setting. The lung injury associated with hyperoxia, ARDS and radiation may be caused by increased local production of damaging oxidants. Therefore, there is interest in increasing pulmonary antioxidant protection. A replication deficient Ad vector (AdCL) was used to transfer the cDNA for the antioxidant enzyme catalase to cultured human endothelial cells for protection against the oxidant stress of hydrogen peroxide[65]. Catalase expression was increased in cells treated with AdCL within 24 hours of administration, and it lasted for up to 1 week. When exposed to $500 \, \mu mol \, l^{-1}$ hydrogen peroxide, AdCL treated cells had significantly improved survival over controls.

Bacterial sepsis is often associated with lung injury and respiratory failure. Endotoxin, released by the bacteria, is felt to be the cause of the lung dysfunction. Endotoxin causes a prostaglandin mediated vasoconstriction of pulmonary vessels, compromising lung function. To inhibit this vasoconstrictive response, cationic liposomes have been used to transfer the prostaglandin G/H (PGH) synthetase gene[66]. PGH synthetase metabolizes arachadonic acid to vasodilating prostaglandins. Rabbits intravenously injected with cationic liposomes containing the PGH cDNA had a marked attenuation of pulmonary vasoconstrictor response after infusion of endotoxin.

SUMMARY

Rapid advances have been made in gene transfer methods of treating human disease. For gene transfer to be of a therapeutic benefit to patients, however, a number of technical problems must be overcome. In the near future, technological advances will improve delivery systems. New methods of gene delivery should have capabilities for targeting the delivered DNA and controlling the level and duration of expression. More importantly, the risk of adverse results needs to be decreased. Intense effort is currently directed toward modifying the immunological response of viral derived delivery systems. To prevent insertional mutagenesis, viral vectors whose insertion is targeted to specific regions of DNA are being developed. Both the technological advances of gene transfer and the information obtained from studying the basic science of disease processes will make the treatment and cure of human diseases with gene therapy a reality.

REFERENCES

1. Lasic DD and Papahadjopoulos D. Liposomes revisited. *Science* 1995; **267**:1275–1276.
2. Hug P and Sleight RG. Liposomes for the transformation of eukaryotic cells. *Biochem Biophys Acta* 1991;**1097**:1–17.
3. Felgner PL, Gadek TR, Holm M et al. Lipofection: a highly efficient, lipid-mediated DNA-transfection procedure. *Proc Natl Acad Sci USA* 1987;**74**:7413–7417.
4. Hazinski TA, Ladd PA and DeMatteo CA. Localization and induced expression of fusion genes in the rat lung. *Am J Respir Cell Mol Biol* 1991;**4**:206–209.
5. Stribling R, Brunette E, Liggitt D, Gaensler K and Debs R. Aerosol gene delivery in vivo. *Proc Natl Acad Sci USA* 1992;**89**:11277–11281.
6. Zhu N, Liggitt D, Liu Y and Debs R. Systemic gene expression after intravenous DNA delivery into adult mice. *Science* 1993;**261**:209–211.
7. Bringham KL, Meyrick B, Christman M, Magnuson G, King G and Berry LC. In vivo transfection of murine lungs with a functioning prokaryotic gene using a liposome vehicle. *Am J Med Sci* 1989;**298**:278–281.
8. Brigham KL, Meyrick B, Christman B et al. Expression of human growth hormone fusion genes in cultured lung endothelial cells and in the lungs of mice. *Am J Respir Cell Mol Biol* 1993;**8**:209–213.
9. Hyde SC, Gill DR, Higgins CF et al. Correction of the ion transport defect in cystic fibrosis transgenic mice by gene therapy. *Nature* 1993;**362**:250–255.
10. Caplen NJ, Alton EWF, Middleton PG et al. Liposome-mediated *CFTR* gene transfer to the nasal epithelium of patients with cystic fibrosis. *Nature Med* 1995;**1**:39–46.
11. Hughes BJ, Kennel S, Lee R and Huang L. Monoclonal antibody targeting of liposomes to mouse lung in vivo. *Cancer Res* 1989;**49**:6214–6220.
12. Glasser SW, Korfhagen TR, Bruno MD, Dey C and Whitsett JA. Structure and expression of the pulmonary surfactant protein-SP-C gene in the mouse. *J Biol Chem* 1990;**265**:21986–21991.
13. Hazinski TA. Prospects for gene therapy in acute lung injury. *Am J Med Sci* 1992;**304**:131–135.
14. Litzinger DC and Huang L. Phosphatidylethanolamine liposomes: drug delivery, gene transfer and immunodiagnostic applications. *Biochim Bophys Acta* 1992;**1113**:201–227.
15. Ross GF, Morris RE, Ciraolo G et al. Surfactant protein A-polylysine conjugates for delivery of DNA to airway cells in culture. *Hum Gene Ther* 1995;**6**:31–40.

16. Ferkol T, Perales JC, Eckman E, Kaetzel CS, Hanson RW and Davis PB. Gene transfer into the airway epithelium of animals by targeting the polymeric immunoglobulin receptor. *J Clin Invest* 1995;**95**:493–502.

17. Plank C, Oberhauser B, Mechtler K, Koch C and Wagner E. The influence of endosome-disruptive peptides on gene transfer using synthetic virus-like gene transfer systems. *J Biol Chem* 1994;**269**:12918–12924.

18. Wu GY, Zhan P, Sze LL, Rosenberg AR and Wu CH. Incorporation of adenovirus into a ligand-based DNA carrier system results in retention of original receptor specificity and enhances targeted gene expression. *J Biol Chem* 1994;**269**:11542–11546.

19. Cotten M, Wagner E, Zatloukal D, Phillips S, Curiel DT and Birnstiel ML. High-efficiency receptor-mediated delivery of small and large (48 kilobase) gene constructs using the endosome-disruption activity of defective or chemically inactivated adenovirus particles. *Proc Natl Acad Sci USA* 1992;**89**:6094–6098.

20. Berkner KL. Development of adenovirus vectors for the expression of heterologous genes. *BioTechniques* 1988;**6**:616–629.

21. Rosenfeld MA, Siegfried W, Yoshimura K et al. Adenovirus-mediated transfer of a recombinant α1-antitrypsin gene to the lung epithelium in vivo. *Science* 1991;**252**:431–434.

22. Rosenfeld MA, Yoshimura K, Trapnell BC et al. In vivo transfer of the human cystic fibrosis transmembrane conductance regulator gene to the airway epithelium. *Cell* 1992;**68**:143–155.

23. Engelhardt JF, Litzky L and Wilson JM. Prolonged transgene expression in cotton rat lung with recombinant adenoviruses defective in E2a. *Hum Gene Ther* 1994;**5**:1217–1229.

24. Bout A, Perricaudet M, Baskin G et al. Lung gene therapy: in vivo adenovirus-mediated gene transfer to rhesus monkey airway epithelium. *Hum Gene Ther* 1994;**5**:3–10.

25. Zsengeller ZK, Wert S, Hull W et al. Persistance of replication deficient adenoviral mediated gene transfer in lungs of immune deficient mice. *Hum Gene Ther* 1995;**6**:457–467.

26. Vincent MC, Trapnell B, Baughman R, Wert S, Whitsett J and Iwamoto H. Adenovirus-mediated gene transfer to the respiratory epithelium of fetal sheep in utero. *Hum Gene Ther* 1995;**6**:1019–1028.

27. Zabner J, Couture LA, Gregory RJ, Graham SM, Smith AE and Welsh MJ. Adenovirus-mediated gene transfer transiently corrects the chloride transport defect in nasal epithelia of patients with cystic fibrosis. *Cell* 1993;**75**:207–216.

28. Wilson JM, Engelhardt JF, Grossman M, Simon RH and Yang Y. Gene therapy of cystic fibrosis lung disease using E1 deleted adenoviruses: a phase I trial. *Hum Gene Ther* 1994;**5**:501–519.

29. Wilmott RW, Whitsett JA, Trapnell BD et al. Gene therapy for cystic fibrosis utilizing a replication deficient recombinant adenovirus vector to deliver the human cystic fibrosis transmembrane conductance regulator cDNA to the airways. A phase I study. *Hum Gene Ther* 1994;**5**:1019–1057.

30. Welsh MJ, Zabner J, Graham SM, Smith AE, Moscicki R and Wadsworth S. Adenovirus-mediated gene transfer for cystic fibrosis. Part A. Safety of dose and repeat administration in the nasal epithelium. Part B. Clinical efficacy in the maxillary sinus. *Hum Gene Ther* 1995;**6**:205–218.

31. Warner B, Wispè J, Yei S, Trapnell B and Whitsett J. Adenoviral mediated gene transfer in the hamster and rabbit. *Pediatr Pulmonol Suppl* 1993;**9**:246.

32. Simon RH, Engelhardt JF, Yang Y et al. Adenovirus-mediated transfer of the CFTR gene to lung of nonhuman primates: toxicity study. *Hum Gene Ther* 1993;**4**:771–780.

33. Brody SL, Metzger M, Danel C, Rosenfeld MA and Crystal RG. Acute responses of non-human primates to airway delivery of an adenovirus vector containing the human cystic fibrosis transmembrane conductance regulator cDNA. *Hum Gene Ther* 1994;**5**:821–836.

34. Yei S, Mittereder N, Wert S, Whitsett JA, Wilmott RW and Trapnell BC. In vivo evaluation of the safety of adenovirus-mediated transfer of the human cystic fibrosis transmembrane conductance regulator cDNA to the lung. *Hum Gene Ther* 1994;**5**:731–744.

35. Curiel DT, Agarwal S, Wagner E and Cotten M. Adenovirus enhancement of transferrin-polylysine-mediated gene delivery. *Proc Natl Acad Sci USA* 1991;**88**:8850–8854.

36. Wagner E, Zatloukal K, Cotten M et al. Coupling of adenovirus to transferrin-polylysine/DNA complexes greatly enhances receptor-mediated gene delivery and expression of transfected genes. *Proc Natl Acad Sci USA* 1992;**89**:6099–6103.

37. Cristiano RJ, Smith LC, Kay MA, Brinkley BR and Woo SLC. Hepatic gene therapy: efficient gene delivery and expression in primary hepatocytes utilizing a conjugated adenovirus-DNA complex. *Proc Natl Acad Sci USA* 1993;**90**:11548–11552.

38. Curiel DT, Wagner E, Cotten M et al. High-efficiency gene transfer mediated by adenovirus coupled to DNA-polylysine complexes. *Hum Gene Ther* 1992;**3**:147–154.

39. Harris CE, Agarwal S, Hu P, Wagner E and Curiel DT. Receptor-mediated gene transfer to airway epithelial cells in primary culture. *Am J Respir Cell Mol Biol* 1993;**9**:441–447.

40. Gao L, Wagner E, Cotten M et al. Direct in vivo gene transfer to airway epithelium employing adenovirus-polylysine-DNA complexes. *Hum Gene Ther* 1993;**4**:17–24.

41. Kay M. Hepatic gene therapy for $\alpha1$ antitrypsin and factor IX deficiency. *Presented at the American Thoracic Society International Conference*, May 1994, Boston MA.

42. Kotin RM. Prospects for the use of adeno-associated virus as a vector for human gene therapy. *Hum Gene Ther* 1994;**5**:793–801.

43. Flotte TR, Afione SA, Solow R et al. Expression of the cystic fibrosis transmembrane conductance regulator from a novel adeno-associated virus promoter. *J Biol Chem* 1993;**268**:3781–3790.

44. Flotte T, Afione A, Conrad C et al. Stable in vivo expression of the cystic

fibrosis transmembrane conductance regulator with an adeno-associated virus vector. *Proc Natl Acad Sci USA* 1993;**90:**10613–10617.

45. Cornetta K, Morgan RA and Anderson WF. Safety issues related to retroviral-mediated gene transfer in humans. *Hum Gene Ther* 1991;**2:**5–14.

46. Miller DG, Adam MA and Miller D. Gene transfer by retrovirus vectors occurs only in cells that are actively replicating at the time of infection. *Mol Cell Biol* 1990;**10:**4239–4242.

47. Hasegawa Y, Emi N, Shimokata K et al. Gene transfer of herpes simplex virus type I thymidine kinase gene as a drug sensitivity gene into human lung cancer cell lines using retroviral vectors. *Am J Respir Cell Mol Biol* 1993;**8:**655–661.

48. Smith MJ, Rousculp MD, Goldsmith KT, Curiel DT and Garver RI. Surfactant protein A-directed toxin gene kills lung cancer cells in vitro. *Hum Gene Ther* 1994;**5:**29–35.

49. Morgan RA and Anderson WF. Human gene therapy. *Annu Rev Biochem* 1993;**62:**191–217.

50. Rommens JM, Ianuzzi MC, Kerem B et al. Identification of the cystic fibrosis gene: chromosome walking and jumping. *Science* 1989;**245:**1059–1065.

51. Sorscher EJ, Logan JJ, Frizzell RA et al. Gene therapy for cystic fibrosis using cationic liposome mediated gene transfer: a phase I trial of safety and efficacy in the nasal airway. *Hum Gene Ther* 1994;**5:**1259–1277.

52. Engelhardt JF, Yankaskas JR and Wilson JM. In vivo retroviral gene transfer into human bronchial epithelia of xenografts. *J Clin Invest* 1992;**90:**2598–2607.

53. Olsen JC, Johnson LG, Wong-Sun ML, Moore KL, Swanstrom R and Boucher RC. Retrovirus-mediated gene transfer to cystic fibrosis airway epithelial cells: effect of selectable marker sequences on long-term expression. *Nucleic Acids Res* 1993;**21:**663–669.

54. Kay MA, Baley P, Zothenberg S et al. Expression of hum $\alpha1$ antitrypsin in dogs after autologous transplantation of retroviral transduced hepatocytes. *Proc Natl Acad Sci USA* 1992;**89:**89–92.

55. Kay MA, Li Q, Liu T et al. Hepatic gene therapy: persistent expression of human $\alpha1$-antitrypsin in mice after direct gene delivery in vivo. *Hum Gene Ther* 1992;**3:**641–647.

56. Lemarchand P, Jaffe HA, Danel C et al. Adenovirus-mediated transfer of a recombinant human α_1-antitrypsin cDNA to human endothelial cells. *Proc Natl Acad Sci USA* 1992;**89:**6482–6486.

57. Canonico AE, Conary JT, Meyrick BO and Brigham KL. Aerosol and intravenous transfection of human $\alpha1$-antitrypsin gene to lungs of rabbits. *Am J Respir Cell Mol Biol* 1994;**10:**24–29.

58. Siegfried W, Rosenfeld M, Stier L et al. Polarity of secretion of $\alpha1$ antitrypsin by human respiratory epithelial cells after adenoviral transfer of a human $\alpha1$ antitrypsin cDNA. *Am J Respir Cell Mol Biol* 1995;**12:**379–384.

59. Nogee LM, deMello DE, Dehner LP and Colten HR. Brief report: deficiency of pulmonary surfactant protein B in congenital alveolar proteinosis. *N Engl J Med* 1993;**328:**406–410.

60. Nogee LM, Garnier G, Dietz HC et al. A mutation in the surfactant protein B gene responsible for fatal neonatal respiratory disease in multiple kindreds. *J Clin Invest* 1994;**93**:1860–1863.

61. Yei S, Bachurski CJ, Weaver TE, Wert SE, Trapnell BC and Whitsett JA. Adenoviral-mediated gene transfer of human surfactant protein B to respiratory epithelial cells. *Am J Respir Cell Mol Biol* 1994;**11**:329–336.

62. Han SK, Brody SL and Crystal RG. Suppression of in vivo tumorigenicity of human lung cancer cells by retrovirus-mediated transfer of the human tumor necrosis factor-alpha cDNA. *Am J Respir Cell Mol Biol* 1994; **11**:270–278.

63. Nabel GJ, Chang A, Nabel E et al. Immunotherapy by in vivo gene transfer in tumors. *Hum Gene Ther* 1992;**3**:399–410.

64. Fujiwara T, Cai DW, Georges RN, Mukhopadhyay T, Grimm EA and Roth JA. Therapeutic effect of a retroviral wild-type p53 expression vector in orthotopic lung cancer model. *J Natl Cancer Inst* 1994;**86**:1458–1462.

65. Erzurum SC, Lemarchand P, Rosenfeld MA, Yoo J and Crystal RG. Protection of human endothelial cells from oxidant injury by adenovirus-mediated transfer of the human catalase cDNA. *Nucleic Acids Res* 1993;**21**:1607–1612.

66. Conary JT, Parker RE, Christman BW et al. Protection of rabbit lungs from endotoxin injury by in vivo hyperexpression of the prostaglandin G/H synthase gene. *J Clin Invest* 1994;**93**:1834–1840.

11

Vertical Human Immunodeficiency Virus Infection

Mark W. Kline

INTRODUCTION

Important features distinguish human immunodeficiency virus (HIV) infection and acquired immune deficiency syndrome (AIDS) in infants and children from the disease observed in adults. Vertical transmission of HIV and the effects of the virus on an immature and naive immune system undoubtedly influence disease expression in ways that as yet are poorly defined. Difficulties in confirming the diagnosis of HIV infection in early infancy, and rapid disease progression in infants with vertically acquired infection, limit opportunities for early therapeutic intervention. In addition, HIV has important adverse effects on the developing central nervous system and normal linear growth and weight gain.

The purpose of this chapter is to discuss some of the distinguishing features of paediatric HIV infection, particularly as they pertain to (1) the epidemiology and pathogenesis of HIV vertical transmission; (2) effects of HIV on the developing immune system of the fetus and infant; (3) influences of age and route of HIV transmission on disease progression and the occurrence of secondary complications; (4) the diagnosis of HIV infection during early infancy; (5) prevention of HIV vertical transmission; and (6) response to therapy and prognosis.

EPIDEMIOLOGY AND DETERMINANTS OF VERTICAL HIV TRANSMISSION

The epidemiology of HIV infection in children is closely linked to the epidemiology of the infection in their mothers. Worldwide it has been estimated that 3.5 million women, most of childbearing age, and over one million children are infected with HIV. About 500 000 children have already developed AIDS. By the turn of the century, four million children will be HIV infected and AIDS will have produced six million uninfected orphans.

The absolute number and proportion of paediatric AIDS cases attributable to vertical transmission have increased as the number of AIDS cases among women has increased. For the 2-year period ending June 1994, AIDS cases among American women increased at an annual rate of 14%[1]. Women accounted for about 17% of all AIDS cases. Since 1992 the number of AIDS cases among American women infected with HIV through heterosexual contact has exceeded the number attributable to injecting-drug use. With a shift toward heterosexual contact as the predominant mode of HIV transmission, many women may be unaware of their or their partner's risk for acquiring HIV[2]. Furthermore, in areas with low maternal HIV seroprevalence rates, ethnic distribution and patterns of maternal risk may differ substantially from those observed in high seroprevalence areas[3], meaning that many HIV exposed or infected infants will fall outside traditionally regarded at risk groups.

Accurate estimates of the total prevalence of HIV infection (as contrasted with AIDS cases or deaths) among women have been difficult to ascertain, but the US Centers for Disease Control and Prevention (CDC) estimates that the HIV seroprevalence rate for women giving birth in 1992 was approximately 1.7 per 1000[4]. It is estimated that about 7000 HIV infected women give birth annually in the United States. With an HIV vertical transmission rate of 20–30%, it is estimated that between 1400 and 2100 HIV infected infants are born each year. Vertical transmission of HIV accounted for 89% of the over 5700 children (less than 13 years old) with AIDS who were reported to the CDC to June 1994[1].

The precise timing of HIV vertical transmission is unknown. There is convincing evidence that infection can occur in utero. The virus has been detected in fetal tissues as early as the first trimester of gestation[5-11], and from cord blood at delivery. Isolation of the virus from amniotic fluid has also been reported[12], but the relationship between this finding and degree of risk for fetal infection is not entirely clear.

Several investigators have detected HIV in placental tissue[13-16], and placenta derived cells can support HIV replication in vitro[17-19], suggesting a pathogenetic role in in utero transmission of the virus. In one report in which serial blood samples were obtained from an HIV infected pregnant woman, the HIV viral sequence obtained from her infant at birth was homogeneous and more closely resembled the sequence population present in the mother's blood during the first and second trimester than it did the sequence population present in the mother at the time of delivery[20].

In addition to intrauterine transmission, there are two other possible routes for vertical transmission of HIV. There is circumstantial evidence in support of the hypothesis that intrapartum exposure to infected maternal blood or genital secretions can result in transmission of the virus. Several investigators have described a virological pattern in infants similar to that observed in primary HIV infection in adults, with no virus detection at birth, peak virus titres between 1 and 3 months of age, and subsequent decline of virus titre[21-23]. Similarly, some HIV infected infants develop new antibody responses to HIV specific peptides[22], or anti-HIV IgM[24] or IgA[25,26] antibody responses in the first few weeks to several months of life, suggesting virus transmission late in pregnancy or around the time of delivery.

A study of twins born to HIV infected women provides interesting indirect evidence for intrapartum transmission of HIV[27,28]. The International Registry of HIV-Exposed Twins studied 115 sets of twins, 23 of which were discordant for HIV infection status (i.e. one twin was HIV infected, the other twin was not). In the discordant sets, first born twins had a 2.8-fold greater risk of HIV infection, as compared with those born second. It is hypothesized that the increased risk of infection observed in first born twins may be related to more prolonged exposure to blood and cervical secretions in the maternal genital tract during labour and delivery.

The relative contributions of in utero and intrapartum HIV transmission to the total burden of HIV vertical transmission are unknown. Recently, an attempt has been made to differentiate the two transmission subgroups based on circumstantial virological findings in the infant[29]. In this proposed scheme, the virus is said to have been transmitted early or in utero if HIV is detected within the first 48 hours of life (e.g. by HIV culture or polymerase chain reaction (PCR)). Late or intrapartum transmission is said to have occurred if virological evaluations during the first week of life are negative, followed by HIV detection between 7 and 90 days of age. Applying these admittedly speculative definitions to published studies suggests that

50–70% of HIV vertical transmission may occur intrapartum[30–32]. In the study of HIV exposed twins[28], the HIV transmission rate for second born infants of caesarean deliveries (the 'in utero transmission rate') was 8%. Subtracting this figure from the overall transmission rate of 35% yields an 'intrapartum transmission rate' of 27%, and suggests that about 78% of all transmission occurred intrapartum.

Postpartum transmission of HIV via breast milk also can occur. The virus has been detected in breast milk by culture[33], and there are well documented reports of transmission of HIV by mothers who acquired the virus postnatally and breastfed their infants[34–36]. The magnitude of the risk of HIV transmission through breastfeeding has been difficult to determine; a review of published studies placed the risk of transmission by a mother infected postnatally at 29%[37]. If the mother had established HIV infection at the time of delivery, the estimated risk to the infant through breastfeeding was 14%.

In the United States approximately 20–30% of infants born to HIV infected mothers acquire HIV infection[38–41]. Worldwide, reported rates of vertical transmission have ranged from about 14%[42] in Europe to 40% or greater in parts of Africa[43].

The factors that determine whether or not HIV vertical transmission occurs are poorly understood. Women with more advanced HIV disease or lower CD4+ lymphocyte counts appear to be more likely to transmit the virus to their infants[43–46]. High maternal viral load has also been associated with a high risk of vertical transmission[47,48]. Infants born prematurely may be at greater risk of acquiring infection[41,43–45], possibly because they have lower concentrations of maternally derived anti-HIV antibodies. Several studies have found that the presence in maternal blood of antibodies to certain epitopes (V3 loop peptides) of glycoprotein gp120 may be associated with a lower risk of HIV transmission to the infant[41,49,50]. However, other studies have failed to confirm this association[51,52]. A role for genetic susceptibility to HIV infection is suggested by the finding that monozygotic twins are more likely than dizygotic twins to be concordant for HIV infection status[27].

Several obstetric factors may influence risk of HIV vertical transmission. Prospective studies from the United States[53] and France[54] suggest that prolonged rupture of membranes may be an important risk factor for HIV vertical transmission. In the French study, the rate of HIV vertical transmission was 30% for mothers whose membranes ruptured more than 12 hours before delivery, but only 17% for mothers with shorter durations of membrane rupture. The mean duration of membrane rupture was approximately 5 hours for mothers who transmitted infection as compared with 2 hours for the non-transmitters. Vaginal delivery also has been implicated as a risk factor for HIV vertical transmission. In the study of twins born to HIV infected mothers, vaginal delivery was associated with a 2.7-fold increased risk of HIV infection in the infant[27]. However, a statistically significant protective effect of caesarean delivery has not been observed in some other large studies of HIV infected pregnant women and their infants[42,55,56].

IMMUNOPATHOGENESIS

The immunological determinants, if any, of vertical HIV transmission are unknown. It has been hypothesized that pregnancy per se may depress maternal immune function, facilitating HIV transmission. Epidemiological data suggest that some viral infections, including poliomyelitis, herpes simplex virus infection and Epstein–Barr virus infection, have a more severe course in the pregnant woman. With respect to HIV, there are conflicting data on whether pregnancy accelerates HIV disease progression in the mother[57,58]. Pregnant women appear to be normal with respect to B and T lymphocyte functions, antibody dependent cellular cytotoxicity, complement activation and cytokine production[59–63].

The naivety of the developing immune system has been invoked as a possible explanation for susceptibility of the fetus and infant to HIV infection and rapid disease progression. The normal neonate is at risk for serious infection because of immaturity in the functions of B and T lymphocytes, granulocytes, monocytes and complement. As a consequence, defences against primary HIV infection and opportunistic infections, as well as immune control of HIV disease progression, are probably impaired.

Destruction of the thymus gland by HIV has been documented in mid-gestation spontaneous abortuses from HIV infected women (Figure 11.1)[16,64]. This early compromise of developing immunity in HIV infected fetuses may lead to a greater than expected rate of fetal loss[16]. The virus can have profound and early effects on the cellular immunity of liveborn infants. As early as 1 or 2 months of age, HIV infected infants have CD4+ lymphocyte counts significantly lower than those of HIV exposed infants who escape infection (Figure 11.2)[46].

Suppression of cell mediated immunity is responsible in large part for the susceptibility of HIV infected individuals to opportunistic

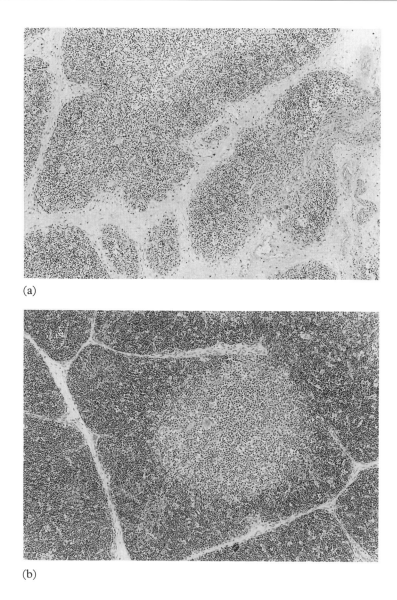

(a)

(b)

Figure 11.1 (a) Thymus gland of mid-gestation fetus infected with HIV. Extensive destruction of normal thymic tissue and passenger lymphocytes is apparent. Nucleic acids of HIV were documented by in situ hybridization (not shown). (b) Normal fetal thymus showing mature thymic cells, Hassell's corpuscles and passenger lymphocytes. (Courtesy of Dr Claire Langston, Baylor College of Medicine.) (Images photographed at ×25, but reproduced at ×15.)

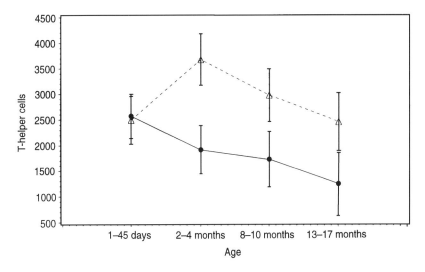

Figure 11.2 Sequential peripheral blood CD4+ lymphocyte counts in infants born to HIV infected women. As with normal infants, HIV exposed infants who escape infection ($n = 28$) display an early rise in CD4+ lymphocyte counts in the first few months of life (broken line), whereas HIV infected infants ($n = 31$) show a blunted rise and significant subsequent decrease in CD4+ lymphocyte counts (solid line) ($P < 0.05$). (From Shearer et al[46] with permission.)

fungal, mycobacterial, viral and protozoal infections. However, HIV can also induce B lymphocyte dysfunction, either as a primary effect or as a secondary effect of dysregulation of T lymphocyte mediated humoral responses and polyclonal stimulation of B lymphocytes by poorly controlled infectious agents. The immunological changes observed in adults and infants with HIV infection are similar, with a notable exception. Lymphopenia and CD4+ lymphocyte depletion are observed less consistently among HIV infected infants than adults, in part because of the relative lymphocytosis of infancy[65,66]. Serious opportunistic infections occur among HIV infected infants with adult normal CD4+ lymphocyte counts[67–69].

CLINICAL MANIFESTATIONS

Only limited information is available on the effects of HIV on pregnancy outcome. It has been reported that HIV infection in the mother may be associated with a greater than expected risk of intrauterine fetal demise, and that HIV can be found in a high percentage of the aborted fetuses[16]. Higher than expected rates of prematurity and intrauterine growth retardation have been observed in studies of infants of HIV infected women in developing countries[43,70-72], but not in most studies of HIV exposed infants in the United States and Europe[38,73]. Most studies that have compared weight, length and head circumference at birth in HIV infected versus HIV exposed, but uninfected, infants have not reported significant differences[38,44,55,56,70].

Infants with vertically acquired HIV infection are usually clinically normal during the neonatal period. A congenital HIV syndrome, encompassing microcephaly, a prominent box-like forehead, flattened nasal bridge, short nose with flattened columella, well formed triangular philtrum and patulous lips with prominent upper vermilion border, has been described[74,75], but its specificity for HIV infection is poor[76].

The CDC AIDS case definitions for adults and children are similar, with several exceptions. Lymphoid interstitial pneumonia and multiple or recurrent serious bacterial infections are AIDS defining only for children. Several other conditions, including certain types of cytomegalovirus and herpes simplex virus infections and toxoplasmosis of the brain, are AIDS defining only for adults and for children greater than 1 month of age[77]. The expanded definition for AIDS in adolescents and adults, which became effective in 1993, does not apply to children (less than 13 years old)[78].

The AIDS case definition is used for purposes of surveillance and reporting. The CDC has developed a separate classification system to describe the spectrum of HIV disease, including HIV exposed infants with undetermined infection status. This system recently has undergone major revisions[79]. The original paediatric classification system included three general categories of HIV exposed or infected infants and children: P0, indeterminate infection; P1, asymptomatic infection; and P2, symptomatic infection. The revised system employs two axes to indicate severity of clinical signs and symptoms and degree of immunosuppression. Clinical categories include N, for no signs or symptoms, and A, B and C, for mild, moderate and severe signs or symptoms. All AIDS defining conditions with the exception of lymphoid interstitial pneumonia/pulmonary lymphoid hyperplasia (LIP/PLH) are included in category C. Several studies indicate that the prognosis of children with LIP/PLH is better than that of children with other AIDS defining conditions. As a consequence, LIP/PLH was separated from the other AIDS defining conditions and placed in category B along with many infectious complications and organ dysfunctions (e.g. cardiomyopathy and nephropathy).

Immunological categories outlined in the revised classification system include the following: 1, no evidence of suppression; 2, moderate suppression; and 3, severe suppression. Degree of immunosuppression is defined on the basis of age adjusted CD4+ lymphocyte counts and percentages.

Use of the revised classification system is relatively straightforward. For example, a 3-month-old infant with *Pneumocystis carinii* pneumonia and a CD4+ lymphocyte count less than $750\ \mu l^{-1}$ has a classification code of C3 to indicate severe signs or symptoms and severe immunosuppression. An asymptomatic 6-month-old infant with CD4+ lymphocyte count and percentage of at least $1500\ \mu l^{-1}$ and 25%, respectively, is classified N1 to indicate no signs or symptoms and no evidence of immunosuppression.

These new clinical and immunological classification categories are mutually exclusive. Once classified, an infant or child may not be reclassified in a less severe category even if improvement in clinical or immunological status occurs in response to antiretroviral therapy or other factors. An infant with HIV vertical exposure and indeterminate (unconfirmed) infection status has 'E' (for vertically exposed) placed as a prefix to the appropriate classification code (e.g. EN1). This designation replaces the P0 classification employed by the old system.

The clinical manifestations of HIV infection in infants and children are varied and often non-specific. Lymphadenopathy, often in association with hepatosplenomegaly, can be an early sign of infection. During the first year of life, oral candidiasis, failure to thrive and developmental delay are other common presenting features of HIV infection.

Table 11.1 lists the most common AIDS defining conditions observed among American children with vertically acquired HIV infection. *P. carinii* pneumonia accounts for about half of all AIDS defining conditions diagnosed during the first year of life[80]; the median age at diagnosis of *P. carinii* pneumonia in children in one series was 5 months[81]. Affected children usually have progressive respiratory distress and hypoxaemia. Fever may be absent. In young infants, in particular, the clinical course may be fulminant. The chest radiograph may demonstrate bilateral interstitial infiltrates, but any pattern of findings, including a completely normal radiograph, can be observed early in the course of illness. Diagnosis of *P. carinii* pneumonia is best accomplished by bronchoalveolar lavage or open lung biopsy.

Table 11.1 Common AIDS defining conditions in children

* *Pneumocystis carinii* pneumonia
* Lymphoid interstitial pneumonia/pulmonary lymphoid hyperplasia
* Recurrent bacterial infections
* Wasting syndrome
* Candida oesophagitis
* HIV encephalopathy
* Cytomegalovirus disease
* Pulmonary candidiasis
* Cryptosporidiosis
* Herpes simplex disease
* *Mycobacterium avium-intracellulare* complex infection

Infants and children with *P. carinii* pneumonia usually are treated with intravenous trimethoprim–sulphamethoxazole or pentamidine. Adjunctive corticosteroid therapy is recommended for adults with AIDS and *P. carinii* pneumonia[82]. Limited information suggests that corticosteroid therapy may be beneficial in paediatric patients, as well[83].

LIP/PLH affects a somewhat older group of children than *P. carinii* pneumonia, with a median age at diagnosis of about 14 months[81]. The onset of LIP/PLH is generally insidious. Cough and tachypnoea often are noted. Examination of the chest reveals few auscultatory abnormalities. Frequently there is marked generalized lymphadenopathy, hepatosplenomegaly and salivary gland enlargement. Digital clubbing may be observed in advanced cases. Chest radiography typically reveals symmetric bilateral reticulonodular interstitial infiltrates, sometimes in association with hilar adenopathy (Figure 11.3). Confirmation of the diagnosis is made by open lung biopsy. Histopathology and immunocytochemistry reveal a mononuclear interstitial infiltrate composed of immunoblasts, plasma cells and CD8+ lymphocytes. The pathophysiology of LIP/PLH is unknown, although Epstein–Barr virus has been implicated as a cofactor in its development[84].

The clinical course of LIP/PLH is variable. Spontaneous clinical remission is sometimes observed. Exacerbation of clinical signs and symptoms may occur in association with intercurrent viral respiratory illnesses. In severe cases of LIP/PLH there is progressive hypoxia and respiratory failure. The management of children with LIP/PLH is largely supportive. Some patients require intermittent or continuous supplemental oxygen. Anecdotal reports suggest that some children with progressive hypoxaemia respond to corticosteroid therapy[85].

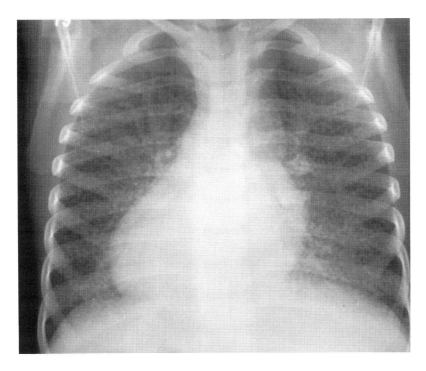

Figure 11.3 Chest radiograph demonstrating bilateral reticulonodular interstitial infiltrates of lymphoid interstitial pneumonia/pulmonary lymphoid hyperplasia.

Bacterial infections occur commonly in children with HIV infection. *Streptococcus pneumoniae*, *Salmonella* species, *Staphylococcus aureus* and *Haemophilus influenzae* type b are the bacteria isolated most frequently[86–88]. Risk factors for bacterial infection in HIV infected children have not been defined precisely, but young children with vertically acquired HIV appear to be at particularly great risk.

The majority of children with HIV infection have central nervous system abnormalities[89–91]. Progressive HIV encephalopathy, which may include developmental delay or regression, spastic weakness of the extremities, microcephaly, seizures and, by computerized tomography, cerebral atrophy and basal ganglia calcification, occurs less commonly. There is evidence that encephalopathy results from central nervous system involvement by HIV itself. The virus has been cultured from cerebrospinal fluid[92], intrathecal synthesis of anti-HIV antibody has been demonstrated[92] and HIV nucleotide sequences have been identified in brain tissue at autopsy[93,94]. Inflammatory lesions, reactive gliosis and white matter degenerative changes are some of the neuropathological findings noted in the brains of HIV infected children[94,95].

Central nervous system infection by HIV is generally restricted to monocytes, macrophages and their derivatives. It is hypothesized that activation of these cells by HIV can result in overproduction of certain cytokines, arachidonic acid metabolites and quinolinic acid, which, in turn, may produce some of the neuropathological changes observed[96,97]. Elevated serum concentrations of tumour necrosis factor (TNF) have been associated with progressive encephalopathy in children with HIV infection[96–98], and TNF can produce white matter destruction similar to that observed in children with progressive encephalopathy[99]. Furthermore, platelet activating factor and products of arachidonic acid metabolism may precipitate central nervous system injury, possibly through upregulation of TNF or other cytokines[97].

A wide variety of other clinical manifestations of paediatric HIV infection have been described. Haematological findings, including thrombocytopenia, anaemia, and leucopenia, are particularly common[100]. Common dermatological manifestations include fungal, bacterial and viral infections of the skin, as well as severe seborrhoeic dermatitis, vasculitis and drug eruptions[101]. Oral findings include infections, aphthous ulcers and parotid gland swelling[102]. Cardiomyopathy, pericardial effusion, myocarditis and cardiac dysrythmias are potentially lethal conditions observed commonly among HIV infected children[103]. Finally, renal disease, with proteinuria, nephrotic syndrome and renal insufficiency, has been reported[104].

DIAGNOSIS

Early diagnosis of vertically acquired HIV infection has important implications for decisions concerning initiation of prophylactic and therapeutic medications, medical follow up, and management of intercurrent illnesses. Unfortunately standard HIV serological tests, including enzyme linked immunosorbent assay (ELISA) and Western blot immunoassay, are not useful in the diagnosis of HIV infection during infancy because of the confounding presence in infants' blood of transplacentally derived maternal antibody. Detectable anti-HIV antibody may persist for 18 months or longer in some cases.

Diagnosis of HIV infection during infancy by physical examination alone is difficult. Generalized lymphadenopathy and hepatosplenomegaly occur commonly among HIV-infected infants, but these findings are neither sensitive (particularly during the first 3 months of life) nor specific for the diagnosis[39].

Hyperimmunoglobulinaemia is a sensitive but non-specific indicator of HIV infection during the first 6 months of life[39]. Some HIV-infected infants, especially those who develop symptomatic disease at an early age, have hyperimmunoglobulinaemia from the time of birth[55,105]; more commonly, it develops over the first few months of life. Because of transplacental passage of maternal IgG, hyperimmunoglobulinaemia G alone is a finding of doubtful significance in the HIV exposed infant.

The assays that have been employed for diagnosis of infection in infancy can be categorized broadly as either direct (detection of virus or viral products) or indirect (detection of host response to the virus). Examples of direct assay methods include virus culture, p24 antigen detection and PCR for detection of HIV proviral DNA. Indirect assays include those which detect intrinsically produced anti-HIV antibodies, such as anti-HIV IgA.

Virus culture is the standard assay to which most others have been compared. In one study of HIV exposed infants 6 months of age or younger, HIV culture had a diagnostic sensitivity and specificity of 80 and 100%, respectively[106]. However, HIV cultures were negative in half of the HIV infected infants studied at birth. Other investigators have reported false negative cultures in up to 50–70% of HIV infected infants tested during the newborn period[30,31]. It has been speculated that this observation reflects low viral burden attributable to acquisition of infection late in pregnancy or at birth. Apparent false positive HIV cultures also have been reported during infancy[107].

Use of p24 antigen detection for diagnosis of HIV infection during infancy has been limited by the generally poor sensitivity of the assay[39,108,109]. Acid dissociation, a technique used to free p24 antigen from immune complexes, may improve the sensitivity of the assay for diagnosis of vertically acquired HIV infection[110–112].

The HIV PCR assay is both sensitive and specific for diagnosis of HIV infection during infancy[106,113–115]. Presumably because of the extreme sensitivity of the assay and cross-contamination of specimens which may occur in the diagnostic laboratory, the usefulness of PCR is limited by occasional false positive results.

Anti-HIV IgA antibody detection has been the subject of conflicting results with regards to its sensitivity for diagnosis of HIV infection during infancy[26,106,116]. The sensitivity of anti-HIV IgM antibody detection, as well as other in vitro assays which detect HIV specific antibody production by lymphocytes from HIV infected infants, is largely unknown[117,118].

Factors other than sensitivity and specificity impact the selection of diagnostic tests for HIV infection during infancy. Although HIV culture has been a useful test in clinical research settings, its more general use has been limited by the labour intensive nature of the assay, the need for a specialized laboratory and equipment, the fact that 2 or 3 weeks are often required for determination of a positive test result, and the expense. It should be noted that test sensitivity and specificity as determined in a research laboratory may not translate to similar findings in the clinical laboratory setting. This fact may apply especially to a test like PCR where meticulous controls are necessary. Because PCR is used to amplify minute amounts of specific DNA by many orders of magnitude, even the slightest contamination can produce false positive test results.

For purposes of clinical decision making, an infant less than 18 months of age is considered HIV infected if he or she is known to be HIV seropositive, or was born to an HIV infected mother, and has positive results on two separate direct tests for HIV (i.e. HIV culture, PCR or p24 antigen detection) performed on separate blood specimens[79]. Cord blood should not be used. An infant is also considered HIV infected if he or she meets the CDC surveillance case definition for AIDS[77].

PREVENTION OF HIV VERTICAL TRANSMISSION

A recently completed randomized, placebo controlled trial of the National Institute of Allergy and Infectious Diseases AIDS Clinical Trials Group (ACTG 076) suggests that zidovudine (ZDV, AZT), given to HIV infected pregnant women and their newborn infants, can reduce the likelihood of HIV vertical transmission[119]. In the study, HIV infected pregnant women with CD4+ lymphocyte counts greater than 200 μl^{-1} were enrolled between 14 and 34 weeks of gestation. Women who had received antiretroviral therapy during the current pregnancy were excluded. The ZDV regimen included three component parts: antepartum ZDV (100 mg orally five times daily), intrapartum ZDV (2 mg kg^{-1} intravenously over 1 hour, followed by a 1 mg kg^{-1} h^{-1} intravenous infusion until delivery), and ZDV administration to the newborn (2 mg kg^{-1} orally every 6 hours for 6 weeks).

Study results indicate that HIV vertical transmission occurred in 25.5% of the mother–infant pairs receiving placebo, but only 8.3% of those receiving ZDV. This represents a 67% reduction in risk of HIV vertical transmission. The drug was well tolerated by both pregnant women and infants. Among infants, the only toxic effect observed was mild anaemia, which was reversible on discontinuation of ZDV.

Because of the design of the ACTG 076 trial, the findings are directly applicable only to women who initiate ZDV treatment during pregnancy (i.e. those who have not had prior therapy with ZDV or another antiretroviral agent) and who have baseline CD4+ lymphocyte counts greater than $200 \mu l^{-1}$. Although serious short term toxicity was not observed, the potential long term toxic effects of ZDV, as used in the protocol, remain to be examined. Ongoing studies are evaluating other strategies for the possible prevention of HIV vertical transmission, including passive (HIV hyperimmune intravenous immunoglobulin) or active immunization (recombinant HIV envelope vaccines) of the pregnant woman and/or her newborn infant.

TREATMENT

Antiretroviral Therapy

As a practical matter, except in the clinical research setting or as prophylaxis against vertical transmission, antiretroviral therapy is rarely initiated in the newborn period. Confirmation of the diagnosis of HIV infection in infancy requires time, and symptoms and signs are rarely present at birth or in the first few weeks of life. Nevertheless, with more widespread use of rapid diagnostic assays (e.g. HIV PCR and immune-complex dissociated p24 antigen detection) it will be possible to initiate therapy earlier. Although there are no controlled studies, strong theoretical arguments favour initiation of treatment as early as possible in the newborn period to suppress early viral replication.

The complex replicative cycle of HIV lends itself to multiple potential sites of therapeutic attack (Figure 11.4)[120]. However, to date, most of the drugs that have been used in children to treat HIV infection (e.g. ZDV, didanosine, zalcitabine and stavudine) are nucleoside analogues that inhibit viral nucleic acid synthesis by binding preferentially to the reverse transcriptase enzyme.

Current indications for antiretroviral therapy include symptomatic HIV infection or asymptomatic infection with abnormal laboratory values indicating significant HIV related immunosuppression. A

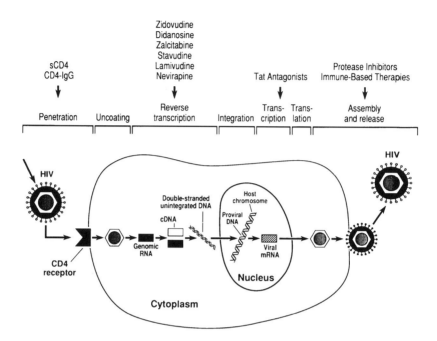

Figure 11.4 HIV replicative cycle with sites of action of some antiretroviral agents. (From Kline[120] with permission.)

CD4+ lymphocyte count of 500 μl^{-1} or less has been used in adults as an indication of significant immunosuppression. In children, determination of immunosuppression based on CD4+ lymphocyte counts is age specific in that normal CD4+ lymphocyte counts are age dependent, with infants having the highest counts[65,66]. Recently, an attempt has been made to define the need for antiretroviral therapy in children, based on age specific minimum acceptable CD4+ lymphocyte counts and percentages (Table 11.2)[121].

The identified toxicities of ZDV in children are similar to those described in adults[123,124]. Dose limiting bone marrow suppression, manifested as anaemia and/or neutropenia, is observed in 30–40% of symptomatic HIV infected children receiving oral ZDV at currently recommended doses[124]. Reported beneficial effects of ZDV therapy in children include improvement in weight gain, decreased hepatosplenomegaly, clinical improvement in HIV associated encephalopathy, decreased serum and cerebrospinal fluid p24 antigen concentrations, decreased frequency of virus isolation and decreased

Table 11.2 Age specific CD4+ lymphocyte counts and percentages indicating a need for initiation of antiretroviral therapy and *P. carinii* pneumonia prophylaxis in HIV infected children

	Criteria for antiretroviral therapy*	Criteria for PCP prophylaxist
CD4+ lymphocyte counts (cells μl^{-1})		
1–11 months	<1750	
12–23 months	<1000	<500
24 months–5 years	<750	<500
6 years or older	<500	<200
CD4+ lymphocyte percentages		
1–11 months	<30	
12–23 months	<25	<15
24 months or older	<20	<15

PCP, *P. carinii* pneumonia.
*Recommendations are derived from reference 121.
tRecommendations are derived from reference 122.

serum IgG and IgM concentrations, as well as transient (about 12 weeks) improvement in CD4+ lymphocyte counts[123,124]. It has not been demonstrated that ZDV therapy in children decreases the incidence of HIV associated mortality or opportunistic infections, possibly because paediatric placebo controlled trials of the drug have not been performed.

Didanosine (2′,3′-dideoxyinosine, ddI) is a useful alternative agent for adults and children with advanced HIV disease and either ZDV intolerance or clinical or immunological deterioration during ZDV therapy. In children, ddI appears to be well tolerated, with beneficial effects similar to those described for ZDV[125]. Pancreatitis has been observed in children receiving high doses of the drug (360 mg m^{-2} day^{-1} or greater). Peripheral atrophy of the retinal pigment epithelium developed in three of 43 children enrolled in one paediatric ddI clinical trial[126]. There were no accompanying changes in visual acuity and the clinical significance of this observation remains to be determined. Unlike ZDV, ddI does not appear to be associated with haematological toxicity.

Zalcitabine (2′,3′-dideoxycytidine, ddC) is not currently approved for use in children. Because of the dose limiting toxicities (e.g. peripheral neuropathy and oral ulcers) described in adults receiving ddC, and the drug's limited central nervous system penetration, it seems unlikely that ddC will be a first line therapy for HIV infection in children. The drug may have a role in combination or alternating therapy regimens.

Stavudine (2′,3′-didehydro-3′-deoxythymidine, d4T) is another agent currently only approved for use in HIV infected adults. However, results of a phase I/II paediatric study of the drug are encouraging[127]. Toxicity attributable to d4T was not observed and most subjects exhibited acceptable growth and stable clinical status during the course of the trial. A multicentre comparative clinical trial of d4T versus ZDV for initial therapy of HIV infected children is ongoing.

Generally speaking, studies of non-nucleoside reverse transcriptase inhibitors (e.g. nevirapine, atevirdine and delavirdine), Tat protein inhibitors, protease inhibitors and other antiretroviral agents have lagged behind development of nucleoside analogues. Nevertheless, paediatric clinical trials of several of these agents are underway.

There are no published studies of combination drug therapy for HIV infection in children. Ongoing multicentre clinical trials are examining various combination therapy regimens. One rationale for using combination therapy is to forestall the development of drug resistance, which has been observed in some HIV infected children treated with single antiretroviral agents[128,129]. Relatively little is known about the impact of HIV drug resistance on response to antiretroviral therapy or HIV disease progression in children. There is evidence that some cases of decreased drug efficacy may be attributable to the emergence of ZDV resistant HIV strains[130]. The potential for vertical transmission of resistant virus isolates, and its implications for therapy of HIV infected infants, remains to be explored.

The long term effects of antiretroviral agents are almost entirely unknown. The potential exists for more pronounced adverse effects on young children who are growing and developing than on adults who have ceased growth. An important multicentre study is examining late outcomes and effects in children who have been enrolled in antiretroviral therapy protocols.

Pneumocystis carinii Pneumonia Prophylaxis

Difficulties with diagnosis of HIV infection during early infancy, as well as determination of significant immunosuppression and risk for *P. carinii* pneumonia, have largely been circumvented by the paediatric *P. carinii* pneumonia prophylaxis guidelines published by the CDC[122].

Prophylaxis is recommended for all HIV-exposed infants commencing at four to six weeks of age. The guidelines state that all HIV-infected infants and those with indeterminate infection status should receive prophylactic therapy until they are at least 12 months of age. Prophylaxis should be discontinued if HIV infection has been reasonably excluded on the basis of two or more negative viral diagnostic tests (HIV culture or PCR), both of which are performed at or after one month of age, and either of which is performed at or after four months of age. After the first year of life, a need for prophylaxis is indicated by the presence of severe immunosuppression (immunological category 3) as defined by the CDC (Table 11.2). Children who have had an episode of *P. carinii* pneumonia should receive life-long prophylaxis to prevent recurrence.

Intermittent (3 days a week) or daily trimethoprim–sulphamethoxazole is generally recommended for *P. carinii* pneumonia prophylaxis in HIV infected children[122]. Daily oral dapsone and monthly intravenous pentamidine are useful alternatives for infants and children who are intolerant of trimethoprim–sulphamethoxazole.

Intravenous Immunoglobulin

Intravenous immunoglobulin (IVIG), given on a monthly basis, can reduce the frequency of infectious complications in some HIV infected children[88,131]. It also has been reported that IVIG recipients have a slower rate of decline in CD4+ lymphocyte counts[132]. This effect appears to be independent of any effect on infection prophylaxis. Unfortunately, despite the beneficial effects of IVIG that have been observed in published studies, mortality rates among IVIG and placebo recipients are similar.

PROGNOSIS

Infection with HIV remains a progressive and ultimately fatal disease, but the time course for development of immunological dysfunction and complicating medical illness is variable and unpredictable for any given individual. In one large retrospective series of cases, the median age at onset of symptoms was 8 months; 80% of patients were symptomatic by 2 years of age[81]. The median age at diagnosis of AIDS for children reported to the CDC is 12 months, but cases have been diagnosed as late as 11 years of age[80]. Early in the HIV epidemic, before the availability of antiretroviral therapy and general use of *P. carinii* pneumonia prophylaxis, median survival times for children with vertically acquired HIV infection were 2–3 years[81,133]. More recent studies suggest that there has been improvement in survival times since the advent of these therapeutic and prophylactic modalities[134–137]. Bimodal expression of HIV disease in children has been noted, with some vertically infected infants having onset of symptoms during the first few months of life, rapid disease progression and early death, and others remaining symptom free or only mildly symptomatic for years[136–138]. Both clinical presentation and age at diagnosis of an AIDS defining condition are important determinants of prognosis. *P. carinii* pneumonia, especially when it occurs during the first year of life, candidal oesophagitis or severe encephalopathy portend a particularly poor prognosis for long term survival[80,81,133,134,138]. It also appears that there are correlations between certain laboratory markers of HIV disease, including low CD4+ lymphocyte counts, poor lymphocyte proliferative responses to mitogens and antigens and lack of anti-HIV neutralizing antibodies, and rapid disease progression[105,136].

A substantial percentage of deaths among HIV infected children occurs in cases where HIV infection is unsuspected until terminal medical illness develops, or an infant's HIV infection status is indeterminate[139]. Prevention of these deaths requires a heightened awareness on the part of caregivers of the risk factors and early signs and symptoms of HIV infection in children, and the application of sensitive tests for diagnosis of HIV infection in early infancy.

REFERENCES

1. Centers for Disease Control and Prevention. *HIV/AIDS Surveillance Report*, 1994;**6**(no. 1):8.
2. Centers for Disease Control. Characteristics of HIV infection among women served by publicly funded HIV counseling and testing services, United States, 1989–1990. *MMWR* 1991;**40**:195.
3. Pratt RD, Hatch R, Dankner WM et al. Pediatric human immunodeficiency virus infection in a low seroprevalence area. *Pediatr Infect Dis J* 1993; **12**:304–310.
4. Davis S, Gwinn M, Wasser S et al. HIV prevalence among childbearing women, 1989–1992. *Program and Abstracts of the First National Conference on Human Retroviruses and Related Infections*, 1993, Washington DC (abstract 27). Washington, DC: American Society for Microbiology.
5. Jovaisas E, Koch MA, Schafer A et al. LAV/HTLV-III in a 20-week fetus. *Lancet* 1985;**ii**:1129.
6. Lapointe N, Michaud J, Pekovic D et al. Transplacental transmission of HTLV-III virus. *N Engl J Med* 1985;**312**:1325.

7. Sprecher S, Soumenkoff G, Puissant F et al. Vertical transmission of HIV in 15-week fetus. *Lancet* 1986;**ii:**288–289.

8. Courgnaud V, Laure F, Brossard A et al. Frequent and early in utero HIV-1 infection. *AIDS Res Hum Retroviruses* 1991;**7:**337–341.

9. Mano H and Sherman JC. Fetal human immunodeficiency virus type 1 infection in different organs in the second trimester. *AIDS Res Hum Retroviruses* 1991;**7:**83–88.

10. Soeiro R, Rubenstein A, Rashbaun WF et al. Materno-fetal transmission of AIDS: frequency of human HIV-1 nucleic acid sequences in human fetal DNA. *J Infect Dis* 1992;**166:**699–703.

11. Lyman WD, Kress Y, Kure K et al. Detection of HIV in fetal central nervous system tissue. *AIDS* 1990;**4:**917–920.

12. Mundy DC, Schinazi RF, Gerver AR et al. Human immunodeficiency virus isolated from amniotic fluid. *Lancet* 1987;**ii:**459–460.

13. Lewis SH, Reynolds-Kohler C, Fox HE et al. HIV-1 in trophoblastic and villous Hofbauer cells and haematological precursors in eight-week fetuses. *Lancet* 1990;**335:**565–568.

14. Chandwani S, Greco MA, Mittal K et al. Pathology and human immunodeficiency virus expression in placentas of seropositive women. *J Infect Dis* 1991;**163:**1134–1138.

15. Mattern CFT, Murray K, Jensen A et al. Localization of human immunodeficiency virus core antigen in term human placentas. *Pediatrics* 1992; **89:**207–209.

16. Langston C, Lewis DE, Hammill HA et al. Excess intrauterine fetal demise associated with maternal HIV infection. *J Infect Dis* 1995;**172:**1451–1460.

17. Maury W, Potts BJ and Rabson AB. HIV-1 infection of first-trimester and term human placental tissue: a possible mode of maternal–fetal transmission. *J Infect Dis* 1989;**160:**583–588.

18. Phillips DM and Tan X. HIV-1 infection of the trophoblast cell line BeWo: a study of virus uptake. *AIDS Res Hum Retroviruses* 1992;**8:**1683–1691.

19. Mano H and Cherman JC. Replication of human immunodeficiency virus type 1 in primary cultured placental cells. *Res Virol* 1991;**142:**95–104.

20. Mulder-Kampinga GA, Kuiken C, Dekker J et al. Genomic human immunodeficiency virus type 1 RNA variation in mother and child following intra-uterine virus transmission. *J Gen Virol* 1993;**74:**1747–1756.

21. Alimenti A, Luzuriaga K, Stechenberg B et al. Quantitation of HIV-1 in vertically-infected infants and children. *J Pediatr* 1991;**119:**225–229.

22. De Rossi A, Ometto L, Mammano F et al. Time course of antigenemia and seroconversion in infants with vertically acquired HIV-1 infection. *AIDS* 1993;**7:**1528–1529.

23. Luzuriaga K, McQuilken P, Alimenti A et al. Early viremia and immune responses in vertical human immunodeficiency virus type 1 infection. *J Infect Dis* 1993;**167:**1008–1013.

24. Pyun KH, Ochs HD, Dufford MTW et al. Perinatal infection with human immunodeficiency virus: specific antibody responses by the neonate. *N Engl J Med* 1987;**317:**611–614.

25. Parekh BS, Shaffer N, Coughlin R et al. Human immunodeficiency virus 1–specific IgA capture enzyme immunoassay for early diagnosis of human immunodeficiency virus 1 infection in infants. *Pediatr Infect Dis J* 1993;**12**:908–913.

26. Martin NL, Levy JA, Legg H et al. Detection of infection with human immunodeficiency virus (HIV) type 1 in infants by an anti-HIV immunoglobulin A assay using recombinant proteins. *J Pediatr* 1991;**118**:354–358.

27. Goedert JJ, Duliege AM, Amos CI et al. High risk of HIV-1 infection for first-born twins. *Lancet* 1991;**338**:1471–1475.

28. Duliege A, Amos CI, Felton S and the International Registry of HIV-Exposed Twins. HIV-1 infection rate and progression of disease in 1st and 2nd-born twins born to HIV-infected mothers: hypothesis regarding in utero and perinatal exposures. *Proceedings of the Ninth International Conference on AIDS*, 1993, Berlin (abstract WS-C10–4). Amsterdam: Congrex Holland.

29. Bryson YJ, Luzuriaga K, Sullivan JL et al. Proposed definition for in utero versus intrapartum transmission of HIV-1. *N Engl J Med* 1992; **327**:1246–1247.

30. Krivine A, Firtion G, Cao L et al. HIV replication during the first weeks of life. *Lancet* 1992;**339**:1187–1189.

31. Burgard M, Mayaux MJ, Blanche S et al. The use of viral culture and p24 antigen testing to diagnose human immunodeficiency virus infection in neonates. *N Engl J Med* 1992;**327**:1192–1197.

32. Denamur E, Levine M, Simon F et al. Conversion of HIV-1 viral markers during the first few months of life in HIV-infected children born to seropositive mothers. *AIDS* 1992;**7**:897–899.

33. Thiry L, Sprecher-Goldberger J, Jonckheer T et al. Isolation of AIDS virus from cell-free breast milk of three healthy virus carriers. *Lancet* 1985;**ii**:891–892.

34. Hira SK, Mangrola UG, Mwale C et al. Apparent vertical transmission of human immunodeficiency virus type 1 by breastfeeding in Zambia. *J Pediatr* 1990;**117**:421–424.

35. Logan S, Newell ML, Ades T et al. Breast-feeding and HIV infection. *Lancet* 1988;**1**:1346.

36. Stiehm ER and Vink P. Transmission of human immunodeficiency virus infection by breast-feeding. *J Pediatr* 1991;**118**:410–412.

37. Dunn DT, Newell ML, Ades AE et al. Risk of human immunodeficiency virus type 1 transmission through breast feeding. *Lancet* 1992; **340**:585–588.

38. Hutto C, Parks WP, Lai S et al. A hospital-based prospective study of perinatal infection with human immunodeficiency virus type 1. *J Pediatr* 1991;**118**:347–353.

39. Kline MW, Hollinger FB, Rosenblatt HM et al. Sensitivity, specificity and predictive value of physical examination, culture and other laboratory studies in the diagnosis during early infancy of vertically acquired human immunodeficiency virus infection. *Pediatr Infect Dis J* 1993;**12**:33–36.

40. Nair P, Alger L, Hines S et al. Maternal and neonatal characteristics associated with HIV infection in infants of seropositive women. *J Acquir Immune Def Syndr* 1993;**6**:298–302.

41. Goedert JJ, Mendez H, Drummond JE et al. Mother-to-infant transmission of human immunodeficiency virus type 1: association with prematurity or low anti-gp120. *Lancet* 1989;**ii**:1351–1354.

42. European Collaborative Study. Mother-to-child transmission of HIV infection. *Lancet* 1988;**ii**:1039–1042.

43. Ryder RW, Nsa W, Hassing S et al. Perinatal transmission of HIV-1 to infants of seropositive women in Zaire. *N Engl J Med* 1989;**320**:1637–1642.

44. European Collaborative Study. Risk factors for mother-to-child transmission of HIV-1. *Lancet* 1992;**339**:1007–1012.

45. Pitt J, McIntosh K, Goldfarb J et al. %CD4 lymphocytes identifies HIV infected maternal risk for HIV transmission. *Program and Abstracts of the First National Conference on Human Retroviruses and Related Infections*, 1993, Washington DC (abstract 28). Washington, DC: American Society for Microbiology.

46. Shearer WT, Rosenblatt HM, Schluchter MD et al. Immunologic targets of HIV infection: T cells. *Ann NY Acad Sci* 1993;**693**:35–51.

47. Roques P, Marce D, Courpotin C et al. Correlation between HIV provirus burden and in utero transmission. *AIDS* 1993;**7**:S39–43.

48. Tibaldi C, Tovo PA, Ziarati N et al. Asymptomatic women at high risk of vertical HIV-1 transmission to their fetuses. *Br J Obstet Gynecol* 1993;**100**:334–337.

49. Rossi P, Moschese V, Broliden PA et al. Presence of maternal antibodies to human immunodeficiency virus 1 envelope glycoprotein gp120 epitopes correlates with the uninfected status of children born to seropositive mothers. *Proc Natl Acad Sci USA* 1989;**86**:8055–8058.

50. Devash Y, Calvelli TA, Wood DG et al. Vertical transmission of human immunodeficiency virus is correlated with the absence of high affinity/avidity maternal antibodies to the gp120 principal neutralizing domain. *Proc Natl Acad Sci USA* 1990;**87**:3445–3449.

51. St Louis ME, Pau C-P, Nsuami M et al. Lack of association between anti-V3 loop antibody and perinatal HIV-1 transmission in Kinshasa, Zaire, despite use of assays based on local HIV-1 strains. *J Acquir Immune Defic Syndr* 1994;**7**:63–67.

52. Halsey NA, Markham R, Wahren B et al. Lack of association between maternal antibodies to V3 loop peptides and maternal-infant HIV-1 transmission. *J Acquir Immune Def Syndr* 1992;**5**:153–157.

53. Burns DN, Landesman S, Muenz LR et al. Cigarette smoking, premature rupture of membranes and vertical transmission of HIV-1 among women with low CD4+ levels. *J Acquir Immune Defic Syndr* 1994;**7**:718–726.

54. Ciraru N, Lefevre Y, Lepage E et al. Obstetrical risk factors in HIV-1 vertical transmission. *Proceedings of the Second International Conference on HIV in Children and Mothers*, 1993, Edinburgh (abstract 22).

55. Blanche S, Rouzioux C, Guihard-Moscato ML et al. A prospective study of infants born to women seropositive for human immunodeficiency virus type 1. *N Engl J Med* 1989;**320:**1643–1648.

56. Italian Multicentre Study. Epidemiology, clinical features, and prognostic factors of pediatric HIV infection. *Lancet* 1988;**ii:**1043–1046.

57. Koonin LM, Ellerbrock TV, Atrash HK et al. Pregnancy-associated deaths due to AIDS in the United States. *JAMA* 1989;**261:**1306–1309.

58. Selwyn PA, Schoenbaum EE, Davenny K et al. Prospective study of human immunodeficiency virus infection and pregnancy outcomes in intravenous drug users. *JAMA* 1989;**261:**1289–1294.

59. Maroulis GB, Buckley RH and Younger JB. Serum immunoglobulin concentrations during normal pregnancy. *Am J Obstet Gynecol* 1971;**109:**971–976.

60. Coulam CB, Silverfield JC, Kazmar RE et al. T-lymphocyte subsets during pregnancy and the menstrual cycle. *Am J Reprod Immunol* 1983;**4:**88–90.

61. Gonik B, Loo LS, West S and Kohl S. Natural killer cell cytotoxicity and antibody-dependent cellular cytotoxicity to herpes simplex virus-infected cells in human pregnancy. *Am J Reprod Immunol* 1987;**13:**23–26.

62. Tedder RS, Nelson M and Eisen V. Effects on serum complement of normal and preeclamptic pregnancy and of oral contraceptives. *Br J Exp Pathol* 1975;**56:**389–395.

63. Yamada K, Shimuzu Y, Okamura K et al. Study of interferon production during pregnancy in mice and antiviral activity in the placenta. *Am J Obstet Gynecol* 1985;**153:**335–341.

64. Papiernik M, Brossard Y, Mulliez N et al. Thymic abnormalities in fetuses aborted from human immunodeficiency virus type 1 seropositive women. *Pediatrics* 1992;**89:**297–301.

65. Denny T, Yogev R, Gelman R et al. Lymphocyte subsets in healthy children during the first five years of life. *JAMA* 1992;**267:**1484–1488.

66. European Collaborative Study. Age-related standards for T lymphocyte subsets based on uninfected children born to human immunodeficiency virus 1–infected women. *Pediatr Infect Dis J* 1992;**11:**1018–1026.

67. Leibovitz E, Rigaud M, Pollack H et al. *Pneumocystis carinii* pneumonia in infants infected with the human immunodeficiency virus with more than 450 CD4 T lymphocytes per cubic millimeter. *N Engl J Med* 1990; **323:**531–533.

68. Kovacs A, Frederick T, Church J et al. CD4 T-lymphocyte counts and *Pneumocystis carinii* pneumonia in pediatric HIV infection. *JAMA* 1991;**265:**1698–1703.

69. Connor E, Bagarazzi M, McSherry G et al. Clinical and laboratory correlates of *Pneumocystis carinii* pneumonia in children infected with HIV. *JAMA* 1991;**265:**1693–1697.

70. Halsey NA, Boulos R, Holt E et al. Transmission of HIV-1 infections from mothers to infants in Haiti: impact on childhood mortality and malnutrition. *JAMA* 1990;**264:**1088–1092.

71. Lepage P, Van de Perre P, Msellati P et al. Mother-to-child transmission of

human immunodeficiency virus type 1 and its determinants: a cohort study in Kigali, Rwanda. *Am J Epidemiol* 1993;**137**:589–599.

72. Bulterys M, Chao A, Munyemana S et al. Maternal human immunodeficiency virus 1 infection and intrauterine growth: a prospective cohort study in Butare, Rwanda. *Pediatr Infect Dis J* 1994;**13**:94–100.

73. Mayers MM, Davenny K, Schoenbaum EE et al. A prospective study of infants of human immunodeficiency virus seropositive and seronegative women with a history of intravenous drug use or of intravenous drug-using partners, in the Bronx, New York City. *Pediatrics* 1991;**88**:1248–1256.

74. Marion RW, Wiznia AA, Hutcheon RG et al. Human T-cell lymphotropic virus type III (HTLV-III) embryopathy: a new dysmorphic syndrome associated with intrauterine HTLV-III infection. *Am J Dis Child* 1986; **140**:638–640.

75. Marion RW, Wiznia AA, Hutcheon RG et al. Fetal AIDS syndrome score: correlation between severity of dysmorphism and age at diagnosis of immunodeficiency. *Am J Dis Child* 1987;**141**:429–431.

76. Qazi QH, Sheikh TM, Fikrig S et al. Lack of evidence for craniofacial dysmorphism in perinatal human immunodeficiency virus infection. *J Pediatr* 1988;**112**:7–11.

77. Centers for Disease Control. Revision of the CDC surveillance case definition for acquired immunodeficiency syndrome. *MMWR* 1987;**36**(1S):1–15S.

78. Centers for Disease Control and Prevention. 1993 revised classification system for HIV infection and expanded surveillance case definition for AIDS among adolescents and adults. *MMWR* 1992;**41**(RR-17):1–19.

79. Centers for Disease Control and Prevention. 1994 revised classification system for human immunodeficiency virus infection in children less than 13 years of age. *MMWR* 1994;**43**(RR-12):1–10.

80. Oxtoby MJ. Perinatally acquired human immunodeficiency virus infection. *Pediatr Infect Dis J* 1990;**9**:609–619.

81. Scott GB, Hutto C, Makuch RW et al. Survival in children with perinatally acquired human immunodeficiency virus type 1 infection. *N Engl J Med* 1989;**321**:1791–1796.

82. The National Institutes of Health–University of California Expert Panel for Corticosteroids as Adjunctive Therapy for Pneumocystis Pneumonia. Consensus statement on the use of corticosteroids as adjunctive therapy for pneumocystis pneumonia in the acquired immunodeficiency syndrome. *N Engl J Med* 1990;**323**:1500–1504.

83. Sleasman JW, Hemenway C, Klein AS and Barrett DJ. Corticosteroids improve survival of children with AIDS and *Pneumocystis carinii* pneumonia. *Am J Dis Child* 1993;**147**:30–34.

84. Andiman WA, Eastman R, Martin K et al. Opportunistic lymphoproliferations associated with Epstein–Barr viral DNA in infants and children with AIDS. *Lancet* 1985;**ii**:1390–1393.

85. Rubinstein A, Bernstein LJ, Charytan M et al. Corticosteroid treatment for pulmonary lymphoid hyperplasia in children with acquired immunodeficiency syndrome. *Pediatr Pulmonol* 1988;**4**:13–17.

86. Bernstein LJ, Krieger BZ, Novick B et al. Bacterial infection in the acquired immunodeficiency syndrome of children. *Pediatr Infect Dis J* 1985; **4:**472–475.
87. Krasinski K, Borkowsky W, Bonk S et al. Bacterial infections in human immunodeficiency virus-infected children. *Pediatr Infect Dis J* 1988; **7:**323–328.
88. The National Institute of Child Health and Human Development Intravenous Immunoglobulin Study Group. Intravenous immune globulin for the prevention of bacterial infections in children with symptomatic human immunodeficiency virus infection. *N Engl J Med* 1991;**325:**73–80.
89. Belman AL, Diamond G, Dickson D et al. Pediatric acquired immuno-deficiency syndrome: neurologic syndromes. *Am J Dis Child* 1988; **142:**29–35.
90. Epstein LG, Sharer LR, Oleske JM et al. Neurologic manifestations of human immunodeficiency virus infection in children. *Pediatrics* 1986;**78:**678–687.
91. European Collaborative Study. Neurologic signs in children with human immunodeficiency virus infection. *Pediatr Infect Dis J* 1990;**9:**402–406.
92. Resnick L, Demarzo-Veronese F, Schupbach J et al. Intrablood–brain barrier synthesis of HTLV-III-specific IgG in patients with neurologic symptoms associated with AIDS or AIDS-related complex. *N Engl J Med* 1985;**313:**1498–1504.
93. Shaw GM, Harper ME, Hahn B et al. HTLV-III infection in brains of children and adults with AIDS encephalopathy. Science 1985;**227:**177–182.
94. Sharer L, Epstein LG, Cho ES et al. Pathologic features of AIDS encephalopathy in children: evidence for LAV/HTLV-III infection of brain. *Hum Pathol* 1986;**17:**271–284.
95. Mintz M and Epstein LG. Neurologic manifestations of pediatric acquired immunodeficiency syndrome: clinical features and therapeutic approaches. *Semin Neurol* 1992;**12:**51–56.
96. Genis P, Jett M, Bernton EW et al. Cytokines and arachidonic metabolites produced during human immunodeficiency virus (HIV)-infected macrophage–astroglia interactions: implications for the neuropathogenesis of HIV disease. *J Exp Med* 1992;**176:**1703–1718.
97. Epstein LG and Gendelman HE. Human immunodeficiency virus type 1 infection of the nervous system: pathogenetic mechanisms. *Ann Neurol* 1993;**33:**429–436.
98. Mintz M, Rapaport R, Oleske J et al. Elevated serum levels of tumor necrosis factor are associated with progressive encephalopathy in children with acquired immunodeficiency syndrome. *Am J Dis Child* 1989;**143:**771–774.
99. Selmaj KW and Raine CS. Tumor necrosis factor mediates myelin and oligodendrocyte damage in vitro. *Ann Neurol* 1988;**23:**339–346.
100. McClain K. Hematologic manifestations and malignancies of children with HIV infection. *Semin Pediatr Infect Dis* 1995;**6:**26–31.
101. Prose NS. Mucocutaneous disease in pediatric human immunodeficiency virus infection. *Pediatr Clin North Am* 1991;**38:**977–990.

102. Kline MW. Oral manifestations of pediatric HIV infection. *Pediatrics* 1996 (in press).
103. Lipshultz SE, Chanock S, Sanders SP et al. Cardiovascular manifestations of human immunodeficiency virus infection in infants and children. *Am J Cardiol* 1989;**63:**1489–1497.
104. Strauss J, Abitbol C, Zilleruelo G et al. Renal disease in children with the acquired immunodeficiency syndrome. *N Engl J Med* 1989;**321:**625–630.
105. de Martino M, Tovo PA, Galli L et al. Prognostic significance of immunologic changes in 675 infants perinatally exposed to human immunodeficiency virus. *J Pediatr* 1991;**119:**702–709.
106. Kline MW, Lewis DE, Hollinger FB et al. A comparative study of human immunodeficiency virus culture, polymerase chain reaction and anti-human immunodeficiency virus immunoglobulin A antibody detection in the diagnosis during early infancy of vertically acquired human immunodeficiency virus infection. *Pediatr Infect Dis J* 1994;**13:**90–94.
107. European Collaborative Study. Children born to women with HIV-1 infection: natural history and risk of transmission. *Lancet* 1991;**337:**253–260.
108. Borkowsky W, Krasinski K, Paul D et al. Human immunodeficiency virus type 1 antigenemia in children. *J Pediatr* 1989;**114:**940–945.
109. Krivine A, Yakudima A, Le May M et al. A comparative study of virus isolation, polymerase chain reaction, and antigen detection in children of mothers infected with human immunodeficiency virus. *J Pediatr* 1990;**116:**372–376.
110. Palomba E, Gay V, de Martino M et al. Early diagnosis of human immunodeficiency virus infection in infants by detection of free and complexed p24 antigen. *J Infect Dis* 1992;**165:**394–395.
111. Miles SA, Balden E, Magpantay L et al. Rapid serologic testing with immune-complex-dissociated HIV p24 antigen for early detection of HIV infection in neonates. *N Engl J Med* 1993;**328:**297–302.
112. Quinn TC, Kline R, Moss MW et al. Acid dissociation of immune complexes improves diagnostic utility of p24 antigen detection in perinatally acquired human immunodeficiency virus infection. *J Infect Dis* 1993; **167:**1193–1196.
113. Cassol SA, Lapointe N, Salas T et al. Diagnosis of vertical HIV-1 transmission using the polymerase chain reaction and dried blood spot specimens. *J Acquir Immune Defic Syndr* 1992;**5:**113–119.
114. Comeau AM, Harris JA, McIntosh K et al. Polymerase chain reaction in detecting HIV infection among seropositive infants: relation to clinical status and age and to results of other assays. *J Acquir Immune Defic Syndr* 1992;**5:**271–278.
115. Brandt CD, Rakusan TA, Sison AV et al. Detection of human immunodeficiency virus type 1 infection in young pediatric patients by using polymerase chain reaction and biotinylated probes. *J Clin Microbiol* 1992; **30:**36–40.
116. Weiblen BJ, Lee FK, Cooper ER et al. Early diagnosis of HIV infection in infants by detection of IgA HIV antibodies. *Lancet* 1990;**335:**988–990.

117. Pahwa S, Chirmule N, Leobruno C et al. In vitro synthesis of human immunodeficiency virus-specific antibodies in peripheral blood lymphocytes of infants. *Proc Natl Acad Sci USA* 1989;**86**:7532–7536.

118. Amadori A, De Rossi A, Chieco-Bianchi L et al. Diagnosis of human immunodeficiency virus 1 infection in infants: in vitro production of virus-specific antibodies in lymphocytes. *Pediatr Infect Dis J* 1990;**9**:26–30.

119. Connor EM, Sperling RS, Gelber R et al. Reduction of maternal–infant transmission of human immunodeficiency virus type 1 with zidovudine treatment. *N Engl J Med* 1994;**331**:1173–1180.

120. Kline MW. Antiretroviral therapy. *Semin Pediatr Infect Dis* 1994;**5**:277–282.

121. Working Group on Antiretroviral Therapy. Antiretroviral therapy and medical management of the human immunodeficiency virus-infected child. *Pediatr Infect Dis J* 1993;**12**:513–522.

122. Centers for Disease Control. 1995 Revised guidelines for prophylaxis against *Pneumocystis carinii* pneumonia for children infected with or perinatally exposed to human immunodeficiency virus. *MMWR* 1995;**44**(RR-4):1–11.

123. McKinney RE Jr, Pizzo PA, Scott GB et al. Safety and tolerance of intermittent intravenous and oral zidovudine therapy in human immunodeficiency virus-infected pediatric patients. *J Pediatr* 1990;**116**:640–647.

124. McKinney RE Jr, Maha MA, Connor EM et al. A multicenter trial of oral zidovudine in children with advanced human immunodeficiency virus disease. *N Engl J Med* 1991;**324**:1018–1025.

125. Butler KM, Husson RN, Balis FM et al. Dideoxyinosine in children with symptomatic human immunodeficiency virus infection. *N Engl J Med* 1991;**324**:137–144.

126. Whitcup SM, Butler KM, Caruso R et al. Retinal toxicity in human immunodeficiency virus-infected children treated with 2′,3′-dideoxyinosine. *Am J Ophthal* 1992;**113**:1–7.

127. Kline MW, Dunkle LM, Church JA et al. A phase I/II evaluation of stavudine (d4T) in children with human immunodeficiency virus infection. *Pediatrics* 1995;**96**:247–252.

128. Husson RN, Shirasaka T, Butler KM et al. High-level resistance to zidovudine but not to zalcitabine or didanosine in human immunodeficiency virus from children receiving antiretroviral therapy. *J Pediatr* 1993;**123**:9–16.

129. Dimitrov DH, Hollinger FB, Baker CJ et al. Study of human immunodeficiency virus resistance to 2′,3′-dideoxyinosine and zidovudine in sequential isolates from pediatric patients on long-term therapy. *J Infect Dis* 1993;**167**:818–823.

130. Ogino MT, Dankner WM and Spector SA. Development and significance of zidovudine resistance in children infected with human immunodeficiency virus. *J Pediatr* 1993;**123**:1–8.

131. Spector SA, Gelber RD, McGrath N et al. A controlled trial of intravenous immune globulin for the prevention of serious bacterial infections in children receiving zidovudine for advanced human immunodeficiency virus infection. *N Engl J Med* 1994;**331**:1181–1187.

132. Mofenson LM, Bethel J, Moye J Jr et al. Effect of intravenous immunoglobulin (IVIG) on CD4+ lymphocyte decline in HIV-infected children in a clinical trial of IVIG infection prophylaxis. *J Acquir Immune Defic Syndr* 1993;**6**:1103–1113.

133. Krasinski K, Borkowsky W and Holzman RS. Prognosis of human immunodeficiency virus infection in children and adolescents. *Pediatr Infect Dis J* 1989;**8**:216–220.

134. Tovo PA, de Martino M, Gabiano C et al. Prognostic factors and survival in children with perinatal HIV-1 infection. *Lancet* 1992;**339**:1249–1253.

135. Thomas P, Singh T, Williams R et al. Trends in survival for children reported with maternally transmitted acquired immunodeficiency syndrome in New York City, 1982 to 1989. *Pediatr Infect Dis J* 1992;**11**:34–39.

136. Italian Register for HIV Infection in Children. Features of children perinatally infected with HIV-1 surviving longer than 5 years. *Lancet* 1994;**343**:191–195.

137. Kline MW, Paul ME, Bohannon B et al. Long-term survival of children with vertically acquired human immunodeficiency virus infection: a proposed definition for use in future studies. *Pediatric AIDS and HIV Infection* 1995 (in press).

138. Blanche S, Tardieu M, Duliege A-M et al. Longitudinal study of 94 symptomatic infants with perinatally acquired human immunodeficiency virus infection. Evidence for a bimodal expression of clinical and biological symptoms. *Am J Dis Child* 1990;**144**:1210–1215.

139. Kline MW, Bohannon B, Kozinetz CA et al. Characteristics of human immunodeficiency virus-associated mortality in pediatric patients with vertically transmitted infection. *Pediatr Infect Dis J* 1992;**11**:676–677.

12

Nitric Oxide Therapy in Infants with Persistent Pulmonary Hypertension

Michael R. Gomez

INTRODUCTION

The Transitional Circulation and Persistent Pulmonary Hypertension

An infant's postnatal fall in pulmonary artery pressure and resistance is the culmination of several associated events of the perinatal period. The fetus begins receiving signals to resorb fetal lung fluid[1,2] and increase surfactant production[3,4] before the birthing process itself. At birth, the baby's first cries fill the alveoli with air and displace the balance of the fetal lung fluid. The simple physical action of alveolar distension causes an initial fall in pulmonary artery pressure[5]. This fall is augmented by other factors as well: the effect of oxygen in decreasing pulmonary artery pressure[6]; and the effects of the long theorized endogenous local compounds[7-10], endothelial derived relaxing factors (EDRFs), that signal the lung vasculature to continue to dilate to accept the full complement of the infant's cardiac output. The shunt pathways of the fetus, the foramen ovale, ductus arteriosus and intra-pulmonary paths, slowly dissipate so that by 3–7 days of age they are nearly absent, and by 8 weeks of age pulmonary artery pressures are nearing adult values[11]. For some infants, however, this normal transition fails to occur for any number of prenatal and postnatal reasons that can be categorized as persistent pulmonary hypertension of the newborn (PPHN) (Table 12.1). The cause of PPHN is as important as the severity of its symptoms because the cause can often be used to predict the outcome of the condition[12]. Those infants in whom normal transition fails and who become critically ill can face a mortality of 20–40%[13], depending on the underlying cause of persistent pulmonary hypertension, the severity of their condition and the treatment necessary for recovery. In addition to high mortality there are significant risks for morbidities, including chronic lung diseases[14], neurological deficits and developmental delays[15] and gastrointestinal disorders, especially related to reflexive suck and swallow[16]. Thus it is paramount that each newborn infant has an optimal opportunity to undergo transition from fetal to adult type circulation as near normally as possible, and minimize those factors known to contribute significantly to morbidity and mortality from PPHN.

Table 12.1 Categories of pulmonary hypertension

Category	Aetiologies
Underdevelopment	Pulmonary hypoplasia (Potter's lung) Congenital diaphragmatic hernia Chronic oligohydramnios
Maldevelopment	Fetal closure of ductus arteriosus Chronic intrauterine asphyxia Meconium aspiration syndrome Congenital structural cardiac anomalies
Maladaptation	Cold stress Hypoxia Hypoglycaemia Hyperviscosity syndromes Sepsis Pneumonia Acute postnatal aspiration syndromes

Intrinsic and Extrinsic Determinants of Pulmonary Vascular Tone

The observation that blood vessels relax in response to an intravenous injection of acetylcholine only when the endothelium remains intact[17] led to the determination that the autoregulatory effect of local vascular bed blood flow is indeed intrinsic. Some years later, Katsuki et al[18–20] performed a series of experiments on the pharmacological activity of a number of nitrate containing compounds. This group noted that nitric oxide gas liberated from these compounds was capable of activating cytosolic guanylate cyclase and raising intracellular levels of cyclic guanylate monophosphate (cGMP), causing profound vascular smooth muscle relaxation. The details of the mechanism of nitric oxide activity, such as its haem dependent activation of guanylate cyclase[21], its extremely short biological half life[22], its inhibition of activity by haemoproteins and methylene blue[23] and its requirement for tissue thiols for activity[24], soon followed. In toto, these findings put forward the notion that the only compound that could share all of these properties is a small, reactive, labile, gaseous molecule present in very low tissue concentrations, such as nitric oxide, and that such a compound could indeed be the determinant of many vascular and biological activities. Together, the observation by Furchgott and Zavadzki[17], that the endothelium was obligatory for vascular smooth muscle relaxation, plus the elucidation of the activity of nitric oxide allowed the unification of the hypotheses that EDRF and nitric oxide could be and were indeed the same compound[25].

HISTORY OF INHALED NITRIC OXIDE THERAPY

Meyer and Piiper reported in 1989 that nitric oxide in extremely low doses (parts per million, ppm) could be safely used in place of carbon monoxide to determine lung diffusion capacity[26], despite some concerns about its toxicity. In fact, several research groups later demonstrated[27–29] that nitric oxide was exhaled in breath, which added further evidence that the compound was indeed endogenously synthesized. These findings supported the idea that exogenously made nitric oxide, given via the respiratory system, might be beneficial in disorders of the pulmonary circulation because it could be delivered directly to the site where it was needed, and its effects would then dissipate rapidly before there were any systemic side effects.

The earliest reports of the use of inhaled nitric oxide (INO) as a selective pulmonary vasodilator were by Archer et al[30] using isolated lungs in 1990, and by Frostell et al[31,32] in 1991, in animal subjects responding to various methods of chemically induced pulmonary vasoconstriction. Shortly thereafter, Pepke-Zaba et al[33] reported the effect of 40 ppm of INO in eight subjects with severe chronic pulmonary hypertension, with ten healthy patients as non-invasive controls. INO produced a significant fall in pulmonary vascular resistance (PVR) without a fall in systemic vascular resistance (SVR).

Moreover, only very small increases in blood methaemoglobin values were measured, confirming its safety in low inhaled doses for brief periods. This study was followed by the simultaneous reports of Roberts et al[34] and Kinsella et al[35] that doses of INO ranging from 6 to 80 ppm given to critically ill near term infants with life threatening pulmonary hypertension and respiratory failure could produce a rapid, sustained improvement in oxygenation without systemic side effects, such as hypotension.

The impact of these reports of improvements in infant oxygenation with INO therapy when there was severe respiratory compromise was immediate, and from them followed a large number of case series, treatment trials and various other clinical trials designed to answer certain pertinent questions about INO therapy. The potential power of INO appeared to lie in its ability favourably to affect only the pulmonary circulation, leaving the systemic circulation intact. A follow up report by Kinsella et al[36] continued to demonstrate that INO could improve systemic oxygenation in critically ill infants, predominantly by relieving persistent fetal type circulatory patterns. This report was followed by a large series of multinational reports of the effects of INO in infants with pulmonary hypertension[37]. In addition, there were reports on INO use in other conditions and in other age groups, such as infants, children and adults with congenital or acquired heart disease, both before and after operation[38–42], pneumonia in patients of all ages[43,44], and in adult respiratory distress syndrome[45]. These reports, in general, were favourable regarding the impact of INO on high pulmonary artery pressure or oxygenation, though some reports of INO failure or a paradoxical response with a fall in oxygenation began to appear as well[46,47]. Short[48] reported at the Workshop on Nitric Oxide in the Perinatal Period convened by the National Institutes of Health/National Institute of Child Health and Development (NIH/NICHD) and the National Heart, Lung and Blood Institute (NHLBI) in December 1993, on series of nine patients referred to her centre for extracorporeal membrane oxygenation (ECMO) with a diagnosis including persistent pulmonary hypertension and respiratory failure (mean oxygenation index of 85 ± 33). All nine patients received INO, and though some showed a transient improvement in oxygenation, all eventually returned to baseline or worsened, and all eventually required ECMO support.

With these initial reports of the successful use of INO, and the summary from the nitric oxide workshop, the focus of the response or outcome to INO therapy shifted from an improvement in oxygenation or echocardiographic criteria of pulmonary hypertension[49] to one of outcomes of treatment with INO. These outcomes included the use of ECMO[50,51], the incidence of death[13], the incidence of significant morbidity, such as bronchopulmonary dysplasia (including length of mechanical ventilation and/or oxygen therapy)[50], or poor neuro-developmental outcome[52]. Economic outcomes, such as cost and length of hospitalization[53,54], could also be compared. The effect of INO therapy on outcomes could then be compared with those of other therapies, such as conventional mechanical ventilation (CMV) and medical therapy[55], or the use of high frequency oscillatory ventilation (HFOV)[56].

The more widespread use of INO revealed occasional circumstances in which it was ineffective, especially when a large component of parenchymal lung disease appeared responsible for the hypoxaemia of respiratory failure. These findings led to more intense scrutiny of the use of INO, namely, its indicated uses and the potential causes for such treatment failures or rare paradoxical responses. Indeed, some of these investigations have led to somewhat contradictory findings that will require more detailed physiological studies.

CONDITIONS AND DRUGS IMPACTING THE EFFECTIVENESS OF INO

Several circumstances that appear to impact the effectiveness of INO have been identified and offer interesting insight into the use of inhaled gas drugs and their ability to access sites of activity.

Lung Volume

Karamanoukian et al[57] reported that in a lamb model of congenital diaphragmatic hernia (CDH), surfactant deficiency decreased lung volume, and was, in part, responsible for the lack of an improvement in systemic oxygenation when these animals inhaled nitric oxide. Largely based on this and similar animal data, there is now support for the routine use of surfactant for the term infant with respiratory failure[58,59], in conjunction with inhaled nitric oxide. Other adjunctive therapy, such as the use of HFOV in infants, has demonstrated its ability to establish a larger functional residual capacity and lung gas volumes than CMV, and safely allow higher mean airway pressures[60]. Thus, HFOV and INO therapy are often used in conjunction to treat respiratory failure. The higher lung volumes set by HFOV, it is speculated, may improve the access to INO to the lung and affected blood vessels. Many ongoing treatment trials and randomized, blinded trials are including both surfactant therapy and HFOV management as variables which may impact the effectiveness of INO. Beyond these treatments is the potential for liquid ventilation techniques to affect lung function and gas exchange, thereby increasing the effectiveness of INO therapy[61,62].

Ventilation to Perfusion Relationships

While there are many reports of improved ventilation to perfusion mismatch upon inhaling nitric oxide, an analysis of a three compartment lung model[63,64] suggests that INO might worsen hypoxaemia, especially by lowering inspired alveolar oxygen concentrations necessitated by using low concentrations of source nitric oxide (<0.1%) and delivering the nitric oxide vehicle, nitrogen. This suggests an explanation for the paradoxical effects seen in response to inhaled nitric oxide[47]. Most reports in animals with smoke inhalation and in babies with other lung injuries noted a general improvement in ventilation to perfusion relationships[65-67], but a few reports in adults[68,69] with respiratory illnesses demonstrated no significant improvements in oxygenation or the degree of venous admixture. This suggests a similar pathophysiology to that seen in infants with respiratory failure and no improvement or a deterioration in oxygenation when inhaling nitric oxide[46,47].

Age

Also of note is the impact of age on the ability of nitric oxide to improve systemic oxygenation. Karamanoukian et al[70] reported that some infants of 2–3 weeks postnatal age, after completing a treatment course of ECMO, had a response to inhaled nitric oxide when they lacked that same response before ECMO therapy. Also, adults appear to respond to INO with a decrease in PVR at a much lower dose (0.1–0.3 ppm)[71] than do infants[34,35]. Whether this effect of age relates to lung volume, to endogenous vascular endothelium nitric oxide activity or to some other factor is currently under investigation.

Other Drugs

An understanding of the cellular level biochemical changes that occur in response to INO has led to other strategies to increase the magnitude and duration of its effect. Intracellular nitric oxide interacts with the guanylate cyclase system and the sarcoplasmic reticulum, producing endothelial cell relaxation. As a result, these systems are prime sites of research for manipulation of intracellular conditions to alter the response to nitric oxide therapy.

Phosphodiesterase inhibitors specific for cGMP could, in theory, have an effect on the action of INO. Silver et al reported[72,73] that the phosphodiesterase inhibitors, WIN 58237 and zaprinast, were able to inhibit the effect of cyclic nucleotide esterification and attenuate cGMP production. Steinhorn and Morin[74] have reported animal research in which such compounds increased both the magnitude and duration of the improvement in oxygenation and fall in PVR in response to INO. The toxic nature of nitric oxide and its metabolites[75] and its short half life[76,77] when exposed to excess ferrous iron in blood make continuous and uninterrupted delivery paramount. Though there have been no reports of tachyphylaxis to INO to date, interruptions in drug delivery can be problematic, with a rapid recurrence of symptoms of pulmonary hypertension and a rapid fall in systemic PaO_2. Experimental phosphodiesterase inhibitors appear to have the ability to increase the magnitude and duration of the response to INO, suggesting that with such adjunctive therapy lower doses of INO could be administered. Furthermore, the lability in the patient's clinical condition would be somewhat less during those brief interruptions in INO therapy for other aspects of pulmonary care, such as surfactant administration or routine airway toilet.

Clearly, the complex relationships involving lung volumes, severity of illness, ventilation–perfusion relationships, age and the effect of other drugs represent critical areas for future investigation.

CLINICAL TRIAL DESIGN

Several large multicentre and single centre clinical trials have been organized to demonstrate the efficacy of INO in the treatment of respiratory failure from pulmonary hypertension. These trials have the common goal of determining if INO is efficacious for the treatment of neonatal respiratory failure from PPHN. However, there is considerable variation among the ongoing trials with regards to the definitions of illnesses, inclusion and exclusion criteria and allowed treatments, as well as in overall study design (Table 12.2). Clinical trial designs have produced much debate as to the appropriate measure of treatment efficacy and study end points. Debated issues

Table 12.2 Summary of active clinical trials of inhaled nitric oxide

	Participating centres	Size	Inclusion	Exclusions	Age/size at entry	Comparison	Placebo	Doses of INO (initial)	End point
Denver NO Study Group	8	288	PPHN by clinical and ECHO diagnosis post-ductal PaO_2 <80	HFOV	≥34 weeks	INO + CMV vs HFOV May crossover	N_2	1–20 (20)	Sustained improvement in PaO_2
Massachusetts General Hospital NO Study Group	5	60	PPHN by clinical or ECHO diagnosis post-ductal PaO_2 <55	HFOV Uncorrected condition CDH Surfactant use	≥34 weeks ≥2.5 kg	NO + CMV vs N_2 + CMV Blinded	N_2	1–80 (20)	OI >40
Boston Children's Hospital	1	100	PPHN by clinical or ECHO diagnosis pre-ductal PaO_2 <100	CDH HFOV Cardiac disease	≥34 weeks	NO + CMV vs CMV Blinded	N_2	1–80 (20)	ECMO or death
NIH Neonatal Network NO Study Group	10	250*	Hypoxic respiratory failure OI >25 May receive surfactant	CDH†	≥34 weeks	NO + CMV vs O_2 (mock) + CMV Blinded	Mock flow	1–80 Repeat trials (20)	ECMO or death
Canadian Inhaled NO Study Group	9	250*	Hypoxic respiratory failure OI >25 All receive surfactant	CDH†	≥34 weeks	NO + CMV vs O_2 (mock) + CMV Blinded	O_2	1–80 Repeat trials (20)	ECMO or death
Ohmeda NO Study Group	>30	320	PPHN by clinical and ECHO diagnosis PaO_2 40–100; MAP ≥10	Surfactant use HFOV CDH	≥37 weeks	NO + CMV vs N_2 + CMV Blinded	N_2	5, 20, or 80 (5), (20), (80)	PPHN sequelae‡
French National Study of Inhaled NO	28	400	Hypoxaemia 20 ≤OI ≥40 All receive surfactant	None	All including preterm infants	NO + CMV or NO + HFOV vs none May crossover	N_2	1–80 (20)	OI at 2 hours >40

CDH, congenital diaphragmatic hernia; CMV, conventional mechanical ventilation; ECHO, echocardiogram; ECMO, extracorporeal membrane oxygenation; HFOV, high frequency oscillatory ventilation; INO, inhaled NO; MAP, mean airway pressure; NO, nitric oxide; OI, oxygen index; PPHN, persistent pulmonary hypertension of the newborn.

*Combined trials (North American Inhaled Nitric Oxide Study).

†Separate, parallel trial.

‡ECMO, death, bronchopulmonary dysplasia, neurodevelopmental delay.

include requirements for blinding and randomization, appropriate end points, entry criteria, types of prestudy treatments, the appropriate placebo and the dose range.

Blinding and Randomization

There is a clear benefit to a blinded, randomized trial compared with a crossover design in demonstrating treatment efficacy. However, some centre history of open label use of INO makes this commitment difficult.

End Points of Therapy

End points of such studies should focus on treatment outcomes, such the incidence of death, the incident use of ECMO (an accepted therapy for conventional treatment failures) and the incidence of certain morbid complications, rather than subjective measures of extra-pulmonary shunting or blood oxygen tension values, which are poor predictors of outcome.

Entry Criteria

Treatment groups vary in severity among these trials because of the wide variation in defining respiratory failure. While some centres have some measure of oxygenation as a criterion (e.g. post-ductal PaO_2 or oxygenation index (oxygenation index = (mean airway pressure $\times$ $FiO_2 \times 100$)/post-ductal PaO_2)), others require additional corroborating evidence of echocardiographic findings consistent with pulmonary hypertension[49,78]. Direct measures of pulmonary artery pressure or resistance in human subjects have only rarely been made in infants[79], and are not routinely used to guide therapy. As a proxy, however, right to left sided shunting across the foramen ovale and ductus arteriosus, along with position of the ventricular septum and velocity of the tricuspid insufficiency jet, all measured by echocardiography, are often used[78]. At best, only a weak correlation exists between any single physical measurement and ultimate outcome. This variation in defining respiratory failure and the criteria for initiating INO may, however, assist in defining those infants who may have a better chance at responding to nitric oxide, or it may ultimately be of no use whatsoever. It may at least allow some latitude in the use of INO and generate more data and experience with less severely ill subjects.

Types of Prestudy Treatments

Certain types of adjunctive therapy, such as exogenous surfactant replacement use[57-59], HFOV[60] and the exclusion of infants with CDH, may be beneficial in narrowing the number of conditions treated and focusing outcome on fewer variables. On the contrary, however, this might also mask important findings. Not all centres, though, support the use of surfactant replacement therapy in term infants or the use of the high frequency oscillatory ventilator. Their use or lack of use appears to be divided along the prevailing philosophy of the study centres as to their roles in the treatment of respiratory failure and their potential for confounding study results.

Choice of Placebo

The issue of placebo has also been somewhat controversial and addressed differently in several trials. The prevailing practical definition of 'placebo' is 'the inert substance or preparation ... with no intrinsic therapeutic value'[80], usually the drug preparation excepting the drug itself, or in this case nitrogen. However, there is a philosophical argument that to reduce the inspired oxygen fractions in critically ill infants in order to deliver placebo is a deviation from the standard of care. It has been argued that the comparison should be between treatment and mock flow or a placebo, such as oxygen, that would not penalize the control group who have no potential to benefit from the trial.

Dose Ranges

A wide dose response to INO has been reported to be progressive[34] to doses exceeding 100 ppm[81] by several investigators. A low dose effect was seen by Kinsella et al at 6–10 ppm[35,36]. Finer et al[37] reported that the dose response for hypoxaemia was largely complete by 20 ppm and that progressively higher doses up to 80 ppm produced no further improvements in oxygenation. Gerlach et al[71] reported an effect of INO on pulmonary artery pressure at less than 0.1 ppm or 100 parts per billion (ppb); however, his findings were largely in adult respiratory failure patients. Depending on the desired effect, the dose can vary widely; however, there appears to be a higher INO dose requirement to improve hypoxaemia than to lower elevated pulmonary artery pressure or resistance. In some groups of infants, the INO dose requirement to relieve hypoxaemia is somewhat higher as well, supporting the speculation that the metabolic response to nitric oxide may vary with endogenous synthase activity, as suggested by Karamanoukian et al[70], or perhaps some other factor[57,67]. Again, there is considerable variation in dosing ranging from an initial dose of 5–20 ppm with ultimate dosing ranging from 1 to 80 ppm.

RECENT DEVELOPMENTS IN INO THERAPY

Use in Infants with Congenital Heart Disease

Neonatal cardiac conditions, such as large ventricular septal defects, truncus arteriosus, atrioventricular canal and anomalous venous connections, can have abnormal PVR at birth and this can quickly worsen with age to a progressive and largely irreversible pulmonary vascular smooth muscle hyperplasia and hypertrophy[82]. The use of chronic, low dose INO can prevent some of the vascular endothelial and muscle changes seen in the hypoxic rat model[83–85]. If true in infants and children with congenital cardiac diseases that have similar vessel changes, INO therapy might prevent vasculature changes that make surgical corrections and postoperative management difficult, and mortality high. For those infants who are not severely ill or are not at risk of developing chronic pulmonary hypertension before their repair, INO could be used postoperatively when high PVR complicates recovery from surgery[38–42]

Use in Premature Infants with Parenchymal Lung Disease

The use of inhaled nitric oxide in premature infants with respiratory distress syndrome (RDS) has been reported by Abman et al[43], by the French multicentre nitric oxide trial group[86] and by Peliowski et al[87]. The infants in each report had somewhat different gestational ages and underlying conditions, and it was difficult to predict responders. The French trial reported a better response to INO when the preterm infants were of a longer gestational age (29–34 weeks) or had echocardiographic findings consistent with PPHN. The infants reported by Peliowski et al[87] all had a history of oligohydramnios and suspected pulmonary hypoplasia. The improvement in oxygenation did not necessarily correlate with survival, and death was not always of a respiratory cause. While these reports are encouraging in a group of infants with few other therapeutic options, clearly carefully designed clinical trials will be needed to elucidate the role of INO for premature infant respiratory failure. Moreover, careful consideration of the use of INO in premature infants should be made, given reports of prolonged bleeding times produced in adult subjects who inhaled 30 ppm nitric oxide[88].

Dosing Considerations

As discussed earlier, there is still wide variability among the data in both the adult[44,45,81] and neonatal[34–37] literature regarding the optimum and maximal effective dose of INO. The general trend and desire is to lower INO doses to as low as possible, while still achieving the desired effect and avoiding potential toxicity. Any excess alveolar concentrations of INO might gain access to poorly ventilated or non-ventilated lung compartments and could potentially dilate areas of shunt[89,90]. This could serve to increase venous admixture and worsen hypoxaemia. Clearly, the lack of clear data in either direction is an argument for careful consideration on a case by case basis for INO therapy, rather than allowing it to become a standard treatment for any condition with elevated pulmonary artery pressures, respiratory failure or hypoxaemia from any cause.

The results of these large clinical trials should offer considerable insight as to the efficacy of INO for PPHN, and define its impact on mortality, the incidence of chronic lung disease and other conditions associated with PPHN. Though no single trial will provide all the necessary or desired information, in combination they should provide considerable evidence to define the appropriate uses and support or refute the effectiveness of INO as a therapy.

NITRIC OXIDE DELIVERY SYSTEMS

With the exception of the short term delivery of anaesthetic gases, delivery of a drug in the true gas phase is relatively unique in medicinal applications. This can produce some interesting and difficult delivery problems. Large concentration dilutions can be made with the current generation of variable area rotametric gas flow devices and gas blenders. However, nitric oxide must be delivered quickly, because of its rapid chemical oxidation in oxygen filled ventilator circuits[91], and carefully, because of its potential toxicity to both patients and health care workers[92–94]. Furthermore, devices designed to measure nitric oxide concentrations, largely borrowed from industrial applications, were not designed to measure nitric oxide in a water saturated, oxygen enriched environment.

Delivery Systems

Variable area needle valved rotametric gas delivery devices are slightly tapered tubes with a float that restricts flow by its position within the tube. These devices are relatively sensitive to pressure and temperature fluctuations and can vary in flow by up to 50%[95]. Furthermore, there can be accuracy problems produced by mixing a fast flowing gas stream from a ventilator with a slow flowing stream from the nitric oxide source cylinder. The use of gas blenders placed in tandem can circumvent some of these pressure effects, but they rely on ratio control, which can be coarse. Furthermore, the nitric oxide must be blended with nitrogen to avoid prolonged contact of nitric oxide with oxygen, introducing yet another source of mixing error.

Newer to medical applications, but with a relatively large industrial experience, are thermal electronic mass flow devices[96–98]. These devices measure the physical property of heat conductance of a gas stream over time, and are thus relatively unaffected by pressure and temperature. Properly calibrated under use conditions, these devices are capable of making large scale gas dilutions very accurately. In tandem, one device could measure actual ventilator (diluent) gas flow, while the other controller could deliver the proper amount of nitric oxide flow to achieve a predetermined nitric oxide concentration. Moreover, because they are electronic, they are capable of electronic feedback control mechanisms that could be developed to adjust gas delivery to changes in diluent gas flow or in response to a change in the clinical condition of a patient. This principle of tandem thermal mass flow control devices, called gas phase titration, is highly accurate and reproducible, and can, in fact, be so accurate as to obviate the need for measurement devices except to serve as alarms or monitors of oxidation products such as nitrogen dioxide[97]. Rapid mixing of the diluent and nitric oxide gas streams can be achieved by placing the mixing site as proximal to the patient as possible, allowing room for adequate mixing of the gas and pre-inhalation measurements of concentrations of both nitric oxide and nitrogen dioxide.

Monitoring

Standard devices for measuring oxides of nitrogen include gas phase chemiluminescence detectors and electrochemical fuel cells. Both methods appear to be reasonably accurate[99–101]; however, they perform optimally when calibrated under conditions exactly like those under which they will be used[102]. Both oxygen and humidity can greatly attenuate the photo signal of the nitric oxide reaction with ozone, the principle under which chemiluminescence operates. This often results in a severe 'quenching' of the nitric oxide and nitrogen dioxide photo signals[103] and underestimation of true values. Equipment redesign to alter converter materials may obviate some of these effects, as can careful calibration of the instrument in water saturated pure oxygen[102].

Electrochemical fuel cells operate by allowing the sampled gas to diffuse into an electrolyte solution or gel, where a reaction occurs which causes a change in the electrical potential of the solution. The voltage change registered by a platinum cathode and silver anode is proportional to the gas concentration. The signal intensity can be altered if inspired gases are water saturated. Changes in the chemical properties of the solution can also be produced when the fuel cells are exposed to high oxygen tensions, which can increase signal strength[102]. Short term studies of electrochemical fuel cell and chemiluminescence analyser performance when placed proximally in the gas flow stream have demonstrated that high oxygen and humidity caused an underreading of actual nitric oxide and nitrogen dioxide values by some 10–12% in chemiluminescence. Oxygen and humidity caused electrochemical fuel cells to overread by about 16%, depending on the brand[102]. Improvements in the understanding of environmental effects on the measurement devices and in the types of devices available[104,105] will ultimately demonstrate their true accuracy and utility, a difficult task in a dynamic system when measuring an oxidizable gas.

TOXICITY CONCERNS WITH NITRIC OXIDE

Endogenous nitric oxide is a free radical gas synthesized in the body by the incomplete oxidation of the terminal guanido nitrogen of the amino acid arginine by a family of constituitive and inducible nitric oxide synthase enzymes[106]. The free electron of the molecule is responsible for the reactive nature of nitric oxide with various compounds[23]. In high oxygen tensions, exogenous nitric oxide begins to oxidize to nitrogen dioxide in less than 1 minute[107–109]. Thus, there must be tight controls on delivery and dosing to minimize this potential conversion. In fact the conversion of nitric oxide to nitrogen dioxide is one of the principal reasons for monitoring inhaled and ambient room gas phase concentrations of oxides of nitrogen. Any method of gas delivery must also have a reasonable means to exhaust exhaled products. With INO, exhaled nitric oxide and nitrogen dioxide released back into the general workplace may pose a hazard to health care workers and visitors, who may be spending 12–16 hours daily at the bedside of an ill infant. Properly designed gas exhaust systems should be able to scrub oxides of nitrogen from the air before releasing them into a closed area, or vent them to a large outside space where they are quickly diluted and pose less danger. In instances where this cannot be assured, ambient room air monitors should be appropriately placed and a safety plan should be developed to deal with exposures. Studies of acute human exposure to nitric oxide have demonstrated that subtle airway and lung injury can occur at 20 ppm[110]. Such brief exposures in lambs, though, were not problematic[31]. Despite the lack of clear toxicity data, both the Occupational Safety and Health Administration (OSHA) and the Environmental Protection Agency (EPA) consider it safe for adults to breathe up to 25 ppm nitric oxide and 5 ppm nitrogen dioxide daily for up to 8 hours, on average, deemed a time weighted average or TWA[111]. Despite these safety limits, rats breathing 2 ppm nitrogen dioxide for 2–3 days, well below the EPA threshold for nitrogen dioxide, developed cilia injury and lung epithelial changes[112]. In humans there exists a potential for cilliary[112], lung[113], alveolar lining protein[114], blood[115] and nucleic acid damage[116] by direct action and by the formation of peroxynitrites[117,118]. Therefore, because of the varied and sparse evidence regarding both acute and chronic human exposure to oxides of nitrogen, it remains prudent to avoid inadvertent exposures. A carefully designed delivery system, scavenging system and workplace can minimize such a possibility. Understanding that exhaled cigarette smoke has up to 600 ppm[119] nitric oxide and NO_x gives a familiar point of reference for exposure effects on lung function.

Exposure to nitrates can also cause methaemoglobinaemia[120], but only rarely have blood concentrations exceeded 5% in infants or adults receiving INO therapy. Patients who repeatedly develop significant methaemoglobinaemia on INO should have their glucose-6-phosphate dehydrogenase and/or methaemoglobin reductase levels measured[121,122]. When other nitrate containing drugs are used concomitantly as therapy for PPHN, careful monitoring of blood methaemoglobin levels is necessary. Should signs or symptoms of toxicity develop, including metabolic acidosis, treatment with intravenous methylene blue[123] or intravenous or oral ascorbic acid[124] should provide prompt reduction of oxidized blood haem. Depending on the patient's clinical condition and response to INO therapy, the decision about whether to continue with INO therapy can then be made.

Until there is a better understanding of the clinical impact of INO therapy and the dangers of both therapeutic and inadvertent exposure to oxides of nitrogen, vigorous attempts should be made to monitor and carefully limit any exposure.

FUTURE DIRECTIONS

Certain difficulties have arisen in testing INO therapy. First, it is highly reactive and unstable in the oxygen diluent gas stream. Both oxygen and nitric oxide are vital as therapy in infants with respiratory failure. Since the gas oxidizes to a toxic product, it must be delivered quickly to minimize toxicity and in order to test its true therapeutic effect. Second, because of its toxicity and reactivity it must be stored in an inert environment of nitrogen and at relatively low concentrations. Though adequate large scale dilutions of nitric oxide in oxygen are routinely made, their accuracy is limited by the technology of variable area needle valved rotametric devices[95] and measurement techniques[99,99–102] and their sensitivity to physical conditions[95,97,102,103,108]. As more information is gathered on the medical application of electronic thermal mass flow control devices, the ability to complete such dilutions should become easier, more reliable and more accurate. Then, higher concentrations of nitric oxide could be resulting in less oxygen dilution with nitrogen, and the true effect of high dose nitric oxide in nearly 100% oxygen could then be adequately tested. Nitric oxide in concentrations of up to 10%, if properly controlled, could be delivered, resulting in much less nitrogen vehicle delivery[97].

The use of chronic low dose INO has been proposed as prophylactic treatment for the chronic pulmonary vascular changes, right ventricular muscle changes and perhaps growth seen in certain types of congenital heart disease[83–85]. While the hypoxic animal model used in these studies does not completely mimic the physiology of congenital heart disease, its potential to prevent these changes is intriguing.

While the short half life, specificity of site of action of nitric oxide and lack of a systemic effect is the appeal of INO therapy, under circumstances where nitric oxide is demonstrated to be therapeutic, a greater dilatory effect of a longer duration might be desirable. Steinhorn and Morin[74] recently reported work on the use of phosphodiesterase inhibitors to do just this, thereby increasing the response to the same dose of INO and the duration of its action by manipulating cellular levels of cGMP. Targeted delivery of INO in the liquid phase, such as via perfluorocarbon ventilation[61,62], would obviate some of the problems of nitric oxide gas exposure with oxygen in sick lungs as a lower concentration could be given to patients, with little leaking into the workplace.

Other, equally exciting areas of investigation of the role of nitric oxide involve manipulation of the system at the enzymatic level. Clearly, the ubiquitous role nitric oxide plays in determining regional and local blood flow is extremely important. Nitric oxide synthase inhibitors, like N^G-nitro-L-arginine (L-NAME) and N^G-monomethyl-L-arginine (L-NMMA), raise systemic blood pressure in animal models of sepsis[125–128]. This makes other manipulations of the nitric oxide synthase system at the gene expression level, enzyme activity level or substrate level an attractive method for redirecting blood flow to favourably affect conditions such as necrotizing enterocolitis, intraventricular haemorrhage and pulmonary haemorrhage.

Careful basic science research coupled with carefully designed clinical trials will surely continue to produce dramatic findings such as have occurred since nitric oxide was first introduced as an EDRF and then inhaled as therapy. Future discoveries will certainly provide a tremendous benefit to infants with disorders of nitric oxide related systems.

REFERENCES

1. Bland RD. Dynamics of pulmonary water before and after birth. *Acta Paediatr Scand Suppl* 1983;**305**:12–20.
2. Bland RD, Hansen TN, Haberkern CM et al. Lung fluid balance in lambs before and after birth. *J Appl Physiol* 1982;**53**:992–1004.
3. Mendelson CR and Boggaram V. Hormonal and developmental regulation of pulmonary surfactant synthesis in fetal lung. *Bailliere's Clin Endocrinol Metab* 1990;**4**:351–378.
4. Dornan JC, Ritchie JW and Meban C. Fetal breathing movements and lung maturation in the congenitally abnormal human fetus. *J Dev Physiol* 1984;**6**:367–375.
5. Milner AD and Vyas H. Lung expansion at birth. *J Pediatr* 1982; **101**:879–886.
6. Corbet AJS and Burnard ED. Change of venous admixture with inspired oxygen in hyaline membrane disease and fetal aspiration pneumonia. *Aust Paediatr J* 1973;**9**:25–30.
7. Ignarro LJ, Wood KS and Byrns RE. Pharmacological and biochemical

properties of endothelium-derived relaxing factor (EDRF): evidence that EDRF is closely related to nitric oxide (NO) radical. *Circulation* 1986:**74**:II–287.

8. Ignarro LJ, Byrns RE and Woods KS. Biochemical and pharmacological properties of endothelial derived relaxing factor and its similarity to nitric oxide radical. In: Vanhoutte PM (ed) *Mechanisms of Vasodilation*. New York: Raven Press, 1988:427–435.

9. Cremona G, Dinh-Xuan AT and Higenbottam TW. Endothelial-derived relaxing factor and the pulmonary circulation. *Lung* 1991;**169**:185–202.

10. Dinh-Xuan AT. Endothelial modulation of pulmonary vascular tone. *Eur Respir J* 1992;**5**:757–762.

11. Clark EB. Heart disease. In: Paxon CL (ed) *Van Leeuwen's Newborn Medicine*, 2nd edn. Chicago: Year Book Medical, 1979:224–239.

12. Riemenschnider TA, Nielsen HC, Ruttenber HD and Jaffee RB. Disturbances of the transitional circulation: spectrum of pulmonary hypertension and myocardial dysfunction. *J Pediatr* 1976;**89**:622–625.

13. Dworetz AR, Moya FR, Sabo B, Gladstone I and Gross I. Survival of infants with persistent pulmonary hypertension without extracorporeal membrane oxygenation. *Pediatrics* 1989;**84**:1–6.

14. Bernbaum JC, Russel P, Sheridan PH, Gerwitz MH, Fox WW and Peckham GJ. Long term follow-up of newborns with persistent pulmonary hypertension. *Crit Care Med* 1984;**12**:579–583.

15. Sell EJ, Gaines JA, Gluckman C and Williams E. Persistent fetal circulation: neurodevelopmental outcome. *Am J Dis Child* 1985;**139**:25–28.

16. Hazinski TA. Current therapy in bronchopulmonary dysplasia. *Clin Perinatol* 1992;**19**:563–590.

17. Furchgott RF and Zawadzki JV. The obligatory role of endothelial cells in the relaxation of arterial smooth muscle by acetylcholine. *Nature* 1980;**327**:524–526.

18. Katsuki S, Arnold W, Mittal C and Murad F. Stimulation of guanylate cyclase by sodium nitroprusside, nitroglycerine, and nitric oxide in various tissue preparations and comparison to the effects of sodium azide and hydroxylamine. *J Cyclic Nucleotide Res* 1977;**3**:23–25.

19. Arnold WP, Mittal CK, Katsuki S and Murad F. Nitric oxide activates guanylate cyclase and increases guanosine 3′-5′-cyclic monophosphate levels in various tissue preparations. *Proc Natl Acad Sci USA* 1977;**74**:3203–3207.

20. Murad F, Mittal CK, Arnold WP, Katsuki S and Kimura H. Guanylate cyclase activation by azide, nitro compounds, nitric oxide, and hydroxyl radical and inhibition by hemoglobin and myoglobin. *Adv Cyclic Nucleotide Res* 1978:**9**:145–148.

21. Craven PA and De Rubertis FR. Restoration of responsiveness of purified guanylate cyclase to nitroso-guanidine, nitric oxide, and related activators by heme and heme proteins: evidence for the involvement of the paramagnetic nitrosyl–heme complex in enzyme activation. *J Biol Chem* 1978;**253**:8433–8443.

22. Ånggård E. Nitric oxide: mediator, murder and medicine. *Lancet* 1994;**343**:1199–1206.
23. Ignarro LJ. Biosynthesis and metabolism of endothelium-derived nitric oxide. *Annu Rev Pharmacol Toxicol* 1990;**30**:535–560.
24. Ignarro LJ, Lippton H, Edwards JC et al. Mechanisms of vascular smooth muscle relaxation by organic nitrates, nitrites, nitroprusside, and nitric oxide: evidence for the involvement of *S*-nitrosothiols as active intermediates. *J Pharmacol Exp Ther* 1981;**218**:739–749.
25. Ignarro LJ, Bugu GM, Woods KS, Byrns RE and Chaudhuri G. Endothelium-derived relaxing factor produced and released from the artery and vein is nitric oxide. *Proc Natl Acad Sci USA* 1987;**84**:9265–9269.
26. Meyer M and Piiper J. Nitric oxide (NO), a new test gas for study of alveolar–capillary diffusion. *Eur Respir J* 1989;**2**:494–496.
27. Gustafsson LE, Leone AM, Persson MG, Wicklund NP and Moncada S. Endogenous nitric oxide is present in exhaled air of rabbits, guinea pigs and humans. *Biochem Biophys Res Commun* 1991;**181**:852–857.
28. Borland C, Cox Y and Higenbottam T. Measurement of exhaled nitric oxide in man. *Thorax* 1992;**48**:1160–1162.
29. Leone AM, Gustafsson LE, Francis PL, Persson MG, Wecklund NP and Moncada S. Nitric oxide is present in exhaled breath in humans: direct GC-MS confirmation. *Biochem Biophys Res Commun* 1994;**201**:883–887.
30. Archer SL, Rist K, Nelson DP, DeMaster EG, Cowan N and Weir EK. Comparison of the hemodynamic effects of nitric oxide and the endothelium-dependent vasodilators in intact lungs. *J Appl Physiol* 1990;**68**:735–747.
31. Frostell C, Fratcacci M-D, Wain J, Jones R and Zapol WM. Inhaled nitric oxide: a selective pulmonary vasodilator reversing hypoxic pulmonary vasoconstriction. *Circulation* 1991;**83**:2038–2047.
32. Fratacci M-D, Frostell CG, Chen T-Y, Wain JC, Robinson DR and Zapol WM. Inhaled nitric oxide: a selective pulmonary vasodilator of heparin–protamine vasoconstriction in sheep. *Anesthesiology* 1991;**75**:990–999.
33. Pepke-Zaba J, Higenbottam TW, Dinh-Xuan AT, Stone D and Wallwork J. Inhaled nitric oxide as a cause of selective pulmonary vasodilation in pulmonary hypertension. *Lancet* 1991;**338**:1173–1174.
34. Roberts JD, Polaner DM, Lang P and Zapol WM. Inhaled nitric oxide in persistent pulmonary hypertension of the newborn. *Lancet* 1992;**340**:818–819.
35. Kinsella JP, Neish SR, Shaffer E and Abman SH. Low-dose inhalational nitric oxide in persistent pulmonary hypertension of the newborn. *Lancet* 1992:**340**:819–820.
36. Kinsella JR, Neish SR, Ivy DD, Shaffer E and Abman SH. Clinical responses to prolonged treatment of persistent pulmonary hypertension of the newborn with low doses of inhaled nitric oxide. *J Pediatr* 1993;**123**:103–108.
37. Finer NN, Etches PC, Kamstra BJ, Tierney AJ, Peliowski A and Ryan CA. Inhaled nitric oxide in infants referred for extracorporeal membrane oxygenation: dose response. *J Pediatr* 1994;**124**:302–308.

38. Roberts JD, Lang P, Bigatello LM, Vlahakes GJ and Zapol WM. Inhaled nitric oxide in congenital heart disease. *Circulation* 1993;**87**:447–453.
39. Girard C, Lehot J, Pannetier J, Filley S, French P and Estsanove S. Inhaled nitric oxide after mitral valve replacement in patients with chronic pulmonary artery hypertension. *Anesthesiology* 1992;**77**:880–883.
40. Haydar A, Muariat P, Pouard P et al. Inhaled nitric oxide for post operative pulmonary hypertension in patients with congenital heart defects. *Lancet* 1992:**340**:1545.
41. Adatia I, Lillehei C, Arnold JH et al. Inhaled nitric oxide in the treatment of post operative graft dysfunction after lung transplantation. *Ann Thorac Surg* 1994;**57**:1311–1318.
42. Berner M, Beghetti M, Ricou B, Rouge JC, Prêtre R and Friedli B. Relief of severe pulmonary hypertension after closure of a large ventricular septal defect using inhaled nitric oxide. *Intensive Care Med* 1993;**19**:75–77.
43. Abman SH, Kinsella JP, Schaffer MS and Wilkening RB. Inhaled nitric oxide in the management of a preterm newborn with severe respiratory distress and pulmonary hypertension. *Pediatrics* 1993;**92**:606–609.
44. Blomqvist H, Wickerts CJ, Andreen M, Ullberg U, Ortqvist A and Frostell C. Enhanced pneumonia resolution by inhalation of nitric oxide? *Acta Anesthesiol Scand* 1993;**37**:110–114.
45. Zapol W and Hurfor W. Inhaled nitric oxide in adult respiratory distress syndrome and other lung diseases. *New Horizons* 1993;**1**:638–650.
46. Barefield ES, Karle VA, Phillips JB and Carlo WA. Randomized, controlled trial of NO for PPHN. *J Invest Med* 1995;**43**(suppl. 1):43 (abstract).
47. Oriot D, Boussemart T, Berthier M, Bonneau D and Coisne D. Paradoxical effect of inhaled nitric oxide in a newborn with pulmonary hypertension. *Lancet* 1993;**342**:364–365.
48. Short BL. INO in neonates referred for ECMO at Children's National Medical Center. *NIH/NICHD/NHLBI Nitric Oxide in the Perinatal Period*, December 1993.
49. Hatle L, Angelsen BAJ and Tromsdal A. Non-invasive estimation of pulmonary artery systolic pressure with Doppler ultrasound. *Br Heart J* 1981;**45**:157–165.
50. Beck R, Anderson GD, Cronin J, Miller MK and Short BL. Criteria for extracorporeal membrane oxygenation in a population of infants with persistent pulmonary hypertension of the newborn. *J Pediatr Surg* 1986; **21**:297–302.
51. O'Rourke, Crone RK, Valenti JP et al. Extracorporeal membrane oxygenation and conventional medical therapy in neonates with persistent pulmonary hypertension: a prospective randomized study. *Pediatrics* 1984; **84**:957–963.
52. Glass P, Miller M and Short B. Morbidity for survivors of extracorporeal membrane oxygenation: neurodevelopmental outcome at 1 year of age. *Pediatrics* 1989;**83**:72–78.
53. Pearson GD and Short BL. An economic analysis of extracorporeal membrane oxygenation. *J Intensive Care Med* 1987;**2**:116–120.

54. Schwartz RM, Willrich KK and Gagnon DE. Extracorporeal membrane oxygenation:Cost, organization, and policy considerations. In: Wright LL (ed) *Report of the Workshop on the Diffusion of ECMO Technology.* NIH/NICHD, US Department of Health and Human Services, Public Health Service, NIH Publication No. 93-3399, Jan. 1993.

55. Wung J-T, James LS, Kelchevsky E and James E. Management of infants with severe respiratory failure and persistence of fetal circulation without hyperventilation. *Pediatrics* 1985;**76**:488–494.

56. Kohelet D, Perlman M, Kirpalani H, Hanna G and Koren G. High-frequency oscillation in the rescue of infants with persistent pulmonary hypertension. *Crit Care Med* 1988;**16**:510–516.

57. Karamanoukian HL, Glick PL, Wilcox DT, Rossman J, Holm BA and Morin FC. Pathophysiology of congenital diaphragmatic hernia (CDH) VIII: Inhaled nitric oxide (NO) requires exogenous surfactant therapy (EST). *Pediatr Res* 1993;**33**:217 (abstract).

58. Kinsella JP, Ivy DD and Abman SH. Inhaled nitric oxide improves gas exchange and lowers pulmonary vascular resistance in severe experimental hyaline membrane disease. *Pediatr Res* 1994;**36**:402–408.

59. Ring JC and Stidman GL. Novel therapies for acute respiratory failure. *Pediatr Clin North Am* 1994;**41**:1325–1363.

60. Meredith KS, de Lemos RA, Coalson JJ et al. Role of lung injury in the pathogenesis of hyaline membrane disease in premature baboons. *J Appl Physiol* 1989;**66**:2150–2158.

61. Leach C, Morin FMC, Fuhrman BP et al. Efficacy and pharmacokinetics of nitric oxide inhalation during partial liquid ventilation with perflubron (LiquiVent™). *Ross Special Conference: Hot Topics '94 in Neonatology,* December 1994, p.162.

62. Wilcox DT, Glick PL, Karamanoukian HL, Morin FC, Fuhrman BP and Leach CL. Perfluorocarbon associated gas exchange (PAGE) and nitric oxide in the lamb congenital diaphragmatic hernia model. *Ross Special Conference: Hot Topics '94 in Neonatology,* December 1994, p. 163.

63. Hansen TN, Corbet AJS, Kenny JD, Courtney JD and Rudolph AJ. Effects of oxygen and constant positive pressure breathing on ADCO$_2$ and hyaline membrane disease. *Pediatr Res* 1979;**13**:1167–1171.

64. Corbet AJ, Ross JA, Beaudry PH and Stern L. Ventilation–perfusion relationships as assessed by a-AND$_2$ in hyaline membrane disease. *J Appl Physiol* 1974;**36**:74–81.

65. Ogura H, Saitoh D, Johnson AA, Mason AD, Pruitt BA and Coiffi WG. The effect of inhaled nitric oxide on pulmonary ventilation–perfusion matching following smoke inhalation injury. *J Trauma* 1994;**37**:893–898.

66. Putensen C, Rasanen J and López FA. Improvement in VA/Q distribution during inhalation of nitric oxide in pigs with metacholine-induced bronchoconstriction. *Am J Respir Crit Care Med* 1995;**151**:116–122.

67. Roz'e JC, Storme L, Zupan V, Morville P, Dinh-Xuan AT and Mercier JC. Echocardiographic investigation of inhaled nitric oxide in newborn babies with severe hypoxemia. *Lancet* 1994;**344**:303–305.

68. Rossaint R, Falke KJ, Lopez F, Slama K, Pison U and Zapol WM. Nitric oxide for the adult respiratory distress syndrome. *N Engl J Med* 1993;**328**:399–405.

69. Bigatello LM, Hurford WE, Kacmarek RM, Roberts JD and Zapol WM. Prolonged inhalation of low concentration nitric oxide in patients with severe adult respiratory distress syndrome. Effects on pulmonary hemodynamics and oxygenation. *Anesthesiology* 1994;**80**:761–770.

70. Karamanoukian HL, Glick PL, Zayek M et al. Inhaled nitric oxide in congenital hypoplasia of the lungs due to diaphragmatic hernia or oligohydramnios. *Pediatrics* 1994;**94**:715–718.

71. Gerlach H, Roissant R, Pappert D and Falke RJ. Time course and dose–response of nitric oxide inhalation for systemic oxygenation and pulmonary hypertension in patients with adult respiratory distress syndrome. *Eur J Clin Invest* 1993;**23**:499–502.

72. Silver PJ, Dundore RL, Bode DC et al. Cyclic GMP potentiation by WIN 58237, a novel cyclic nucleotide phosphodiesterase inhibitor. *J Pharmacol Exp Ther* 1994;**271**:1143–1149.

73. Dundore RL, Claes DM, Wheeler LT et al. Zaprinast increases cyclic GMP levels in plasma and aortic tissue of rats. *Eur J Pharmacol* 1993;**249**:293–297.

74. Steinhorn RH and Morin FC. The use of phosphodiesterase inhibitors with inhaled nitric oxide in animals. *Ross Special Conference: Hot Topics '94 in Neonatology*, December 1994, p. 12.

75. Freeman B. Free radical chemistry of nitric oxide. Looking at the dark side. *Chest* 1994;**105**(Suppl.):79–84S.

76. Kiechle FL and Malinski T. Nitric oxide. Biochemistry, pathophysiology, and detection. *Am J Clin Pathol* 1993;**249**:567–575.

77. Oda H, Nogami H and Nakajima T. Reaction of hemoglobin with nitric oxide and nitrogen dioxide in mice. *J Toxicol Environ Health* 1980;**6**:673–678.

78. Oberhensli I, Braden G, Girod M and Friedli B. Estimation of pulmonary artery pressure by ultrasound. A study comparing simultaneously recorded pulmonary valve echogram and pulmonary artery pressures. *Pediatr Cardiol* 1982;**2**:123–130.

79. Gersony WM. Neonatal pulmonary hypertension: pathophysiology, classification and etiology. *Clin Perinatol* 1984;**11**:517–524.

80. Friel JP (ed). *Dorland's Illustrated Medical Dictionary*, 26th edn. Philadelphia: Saunders, 1981.

81. Young WJ, Brampton JD and Finfer SR. Inhaled nitric oxide in acute respiratory failure in adults. *Br J Anesth* 1994;**73**:499–502.

82. Rabinovich M. Vascular pathology of PPHNS. In: Long WA (ed) *Fetal and Neonatal Cardiology*. Philadelphia: Saunders, 1990:656–666.

83. Kouyoumdjian C, Adnot S, Lavame M, Eddahibi S, Bousbaa H and Raffestin B. Continuous inhalation of nitric oxide protects against the development of pulmonary hypertension in chronically hypoxic rats. *J Clin Invest* 1994;**94**:578–584.

84. Roberts JD. New directions in nitric oxide research. *Ross Special Conference: Hot Topics '94 in Neonatolgy*, December 1994, pp. 281–287.

85. Roberts JD, Roberts CT, Jones RC, Zapol WM and Bloch KD. Continuous nitric oxide inhalation reduces pulmonary arterial structural changes, right ventricular hypertrophy, and growth retardation in the hypoxic newborn rat. *Circ Res* 1995;**76:**215–222.

86. Lacaze-Masmontiel T. Inhaled nitric oxide in severely hypoxemic newborns: the preliminary French experience. *Ross Special Conference: Hot Topics '94 in Neonatology*, December 1994, pp. 277–280.

87. Peliowski A, Finer NN, Etches PC, Tierney AJ and Ryan CA. Inhaled nitric oxide for preterm infants with prolonged rupture of membranes. *J Pediatr* 1995;**126:**450–453.

88. Hogman M, Frostell C, Arnberg H and Hedensiernia G. Bleeding time prolongation and nitric oxide inhalation. *Lancet* 1993;**341:**1664–1665.

89. Rovira I, Chen T-Y, Winkler M, Kawai N, Bloch KD and Zapol WM. Effects of inhaled nitric oxide on pulmonary hemodynamics and gas exchange. *J Appl Physiol* 1994;**76:**345–355.

90. Bigatello LM, Hurford WE, Kacmarek RM, Roberts JD and Zapol WM. Inhaled nitric oxide is a selective pulmonary vasodilator in septic patients with ARDS. *Am Rev Respir Dis* 1992;**145**(suppl.):185 (abstract).

91. Motsch J, Weiman J, Fresenius M, Gagel K and Martin E. [In vitro study of the formation of NO_2 in inhalation nitrogen monoxide.] *Anesthesiol Intensivmed Noffalmed Schmerzther* 1994;**29:**157–162.

92. Kagawa J. Evaluation of biologic significance of nitrogen oxide exposure. *Tokai J Exp Clin Med* 1985;**10:**348–353.

93. Gustafsson LE. Experimental studies on nitric oxide. *Scand J Work Environ Health* 1993;**19**(suppl. 2):44–49.

94. Wennmalm A, Benthin G, Edlund A et al. Metabolism and excretion of nitric oxide in humans. An experimental and clinical study. *Circ Res* 1993;**73:**1121–1127.

95. Cusick CF (ed). *Flow Meter Engineering Handbook*, 5th edn. Fort Washington PA: Honeywell Inc., Process Control Division, 1977.

96. Young JD. A universal nitric oxide delivery system. *Br J Anesth* 1994;**73:**700–702.

97. Gomez MR. Nitric oxide delivery devices. *NIH/NICHD/NHLBI Nitric Oxide in the Perinatal Period*, December 1993.

98. Watkins DN, Jenkins IR, Rankin JM and Clark GM. Inhaled nitric oxide in severe acute respiratory failure – its use in intensive care and description of a delivery system. *Anesth Intensive Care* 1993;**21:**661–666.

99. Henneberg SW, Jensen SB, Jensen EW and Andersen PK. [Inhalation therapy with nitric oxide – an evaluation of a dosage system and clinical examples.] *Ugeskr Laeger* 1994;**156:**4245–4250.

100. Petros AJ, Cox PB and Bohn D. A simple method for monitoring concentration of inhaled nitric oxide. *Lancet* 1992;**340:**1167.

101. Noguchi T, Miyakawa H, Mori M et al. [Evaluation of a new nitric oxide delivery system during mechanical ventilation.] *Masui* 1994;**43:**1083–1086.

102. Gomez MR, Moon JK and Jarriel WS. Evaluation of a dynamic system for delivery of nitric oxide for the treatment of persistent pulmonary hypertension (PPHN). *Pediatr Res* 1994;**35**:334 (abstract).

103. Thermo Environmental Instruments, Inc., Franklin, MA. *Quenching and viscosity effects on NO–NO$_2$–NO$_x$ chemiluminescence measurements*, TP-42-01. 29 October 1993.

104. Tsukahara H, Gordienko DV and Goligorsky MS. Continuous monitoring of nitric oxide release from human umbilical vein endothelial cells. *Biochem Biophys Res Commun* 1993;**193**:722–729.

105. Taha Z, Kiechle F and Malinski T. Oxidation of nitric oxide in oxygen in biological systems monitored by porphyrinic sensor. *Biochem Biophys Res Commun* 1992;**188**:734–739.

106. Sessa WC. The nitric oxide synthase family of proteins. *J Vasc Res* 1994;**31**:131–143.

107. Stamler JS, Singel DJ and Loscalzo J. Biochemistry of nitric oxide and its redox-activated forms. *Science* 1992;**258**:1898–1902.

108. Miyamoto K, Aida A, Nishimura M et al. Effects of humidity and temperature on nitrogen dioxide formation from nitric oxide. *Lancet* 1994; **343**:1099–1100.

109. Bouchet M, Renaudin MH, Reveau C, Mercier JC, Dehan M and Zupan V. Safety requirements for use of inhaled nitric oxide in neonates. *Lancet* 1993;**341**:968–969.

110. von Nieding G, Wagner HM and Krekeler H. Investigation of the acute effects of nitrogen monoxide on lung function in man. *Proceedings of the Third International Clean Air Congress*, 1973:A14–16.

111. Centers for Disease Control. National Institute for Occupational Safety and Health: recommendations for occupational safety and health standards. *MMWR* 1988;**37**(suppl. 17):1–29.

112. Stephens RJ, Freeman G and Evans MJ. Early response of lungs to low levels of nitrogen dioxide. *Arch Environ Health* 1972;**24**:160–179.

113. Stavert DM and Lehnert BE. Nitrogen oxides and nitrogen dioxide as inducers of acute pulmonary injury when inhaled at relatively high concentrations for brief periods. *Inhalational Toxicol* 1990;**2**:53–67.

114. Haddad IY, Pataki G, Hu P, Galliani C, Beckman JS and Metalon S. Quantitation of nitrotyrosine levels in lung secretions of patients and animals with acute lung injury. *J Clin Invest* 1994;**94**:2407–2413.

115. Kinsella JP and Abman SH. Methemoglobin during nitric oxide therapy with high frequency ventilator. *Lancet* 1993;**342**:615.

116. Nguyen T, Brunson D, Crespi CL, Penman BW, Wishnok JS and Tannenbaum SR. DNA damage and mutation of human cells exposed to nitric oxide in vitro. *Proc Natl Acad Sci USA* 1992;**89**:3030–3034.

117. Beckman JS. Peroxynitrite versus hydroxyl radical: the role of nitric oxide in superoxide dependent cerebral injury. *Ann NY Acad Sci* 1994;**738**:69–75.

118. Radi R, Beckman JS, Bush KM and Freeman BA. Peroxynitrite oxidation of sulfhydryls. *J Biol Chem* 1991;**266**:4244–4250.

119. Cueto R and Pryor WA. Cigarette smoke chemistry: conversion of nitric oxide to nitrogen dioxide and reaction of nitrogen oxides and other smoke components as studied by Fourier transformation infared spectroscopy. *Vibrational Spectrosc* 1994;7:97–111.

120. Dusdicker LB, Getchell JP, Liarakos TM, Hausler WJ and Dungy CI. Nitrate in baby foods. Adding to the nitrate mosaic. *Arch Pediatr Adolesc Med* 1994;**148**:490–494.

121. Ogata M, Ishii K, Ioku N and Meguro T. Methemoglobin formation in the blood of Japanese subjects and mice suffering from acatalasemia in response to methemoglobin inducers. *Physiol Chem Phys Med NMR* 1990;**22**:125–134.

122. Wessel DL, Adatia I, Thompson JE and Hickey PR. Delivery and monitoring inhaled nitric oxide in patients with pulmonary hypertension. *Crit Care Med* 1994;**22**:930–938.

123. Buenger JW and Mauro VF. Organic nitrate-induced methemoglobinemia. *DICP* 1989;**23**:283–288.

124. Schott AM, Gozzo I, Chareyre S and Delmas PD. Flutamide-induced methemoglobinemia. *DICP* 1991;**25**:600–601.

125. Petros A, Bennett D and Vallance P. Effect of nitric oxide synthase inhibitors on hypotension in patients with septic shock. *Lancet* 1991; **338**:1557–1558.

126. Wright CE, Rees DD and Moncada S. Protective and pathological roles of nitric oxide in endotoxic shock. *Cardiovasc Res* 1992;**26**:48–57.

127. Nava E, Palmer PM and Moncada S. The role of nitric oxide in endotoxic shock: effects of N^G-monomethyl-L-arginine. *J Cardiovasc Pharmacol* 1992;**20**(suppl. 12):S132–134.

128. Booke M, Meyer J, Linghau W, Hinder F, Traber L and Traber DL. Use of nitric oxide synthase inhibitors in animal models of sepsis. *New Horizons* 1995;**3**:123–138.

Index

Note: tables in **bold**, figures in *italic*.